UNDERSTANDING

EQUINE
PREVENTIVE
MEDICINE

YOUR **GUIDE** TO HORSE HEALTH
CARE AND MANAGEMENT

UNDERSTANDING

EQUINE
PREVENTIVE
MEDICINE

YOUR **GUIDE** TO HORSE HEALTH
CARE AND MANAGEMENT

By Bradford G. Bentz, VMD, MS

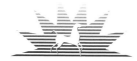

The Blood-Horse, Inc. Lexington, KY

ISBN 1-58150-086-6

Library of Congress Control Number: 2002101454

Printed in the United States of America

First Edition: October 2002

1 2 3 4 5 6 7 8 9 10

Contents

CHAPTER 1

Principles of Disease Prevention

Programs to control infectious disease in individual horses and groups of horses are necessary to maximize health and performance. Prevention programs extend beyond vaccination and deworming and include plans for sudden outbreaks of disease and management of horses with health problems. Having a good preventive care program ultimately can save an owner time and money.

Infectious disease occurs when infectious agents overcome inherent protection in an individual or group. A successful prevention program must, therefore, reduce the rates of exposure of the horse(s) to infectious agents and maximize resistance against such agents. The incidence of infectious disease in a given horse population rises with increased numbers of individuals, concentration of susceptible horses at the facility, movement of new horses into and out of the facility, and environmental and management factors that favor an infectious disease's development and transmission.

On breeding farms, continually adding and mixing horses of various ages and from various locations, plus a resident high proportion of susceptible young horses and pregnant mares, heightens the risk for the introduction and transmission of infectious diseases. Separating horses by age and function can minimize the inherent risks in such situations. Mares and foals should be separated from weanlings, yearlings, horses in training, and transient mares.

Show barns and racetracks are conducive to the introduction and perpetuation of infectious diseases among the resident horses. Any new horse entering one of these facilities (including breeding farms) should have a negative Coggins test and documentation of timely vaccination and deworming. Newly arriving animals should be quarantined for two to four weeks. The farm veterinarian should oversee the quarantined horses and continually and concurrently evaluate these horses for signs or symptoms of infectious disease. Any horse(s) with an infectious disease should be isolated, preferably in a separate facility. Because isolation is frequently impossible, the horse(s) should be placed in a location that minimizes exposure to other animals, common water sources, and shared ventilation. Buckets and feeders, grooming implements, tools, and any

> ## AT A GLANCE
>
> • A successful prevention program reduces horses' risks of exposure to infectious agents.
>
> • Separating horses by age and function can minimize inherent risks.
>
> • Quarantine newly arriving animals; isolate horses with an infectious disease.

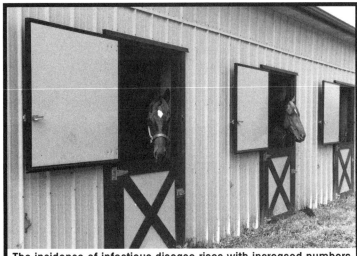

The incidence of infectious disease rises with increased numbers and concentration of individuals.

other items exposed to the infectious animal or to its stall should be used only for that animal. Strict isolation protocol mandates that all other horses be cared for first or by separate farm personnel before the diseased animal receives care. This minimizes potential contact with non-diseased animals by farm personnel who have handled the infectious horses and/or items used to tend to them. Wearing boots, coveralls, and gloves, and then strict disinfection of these garments and hands are necessary after workers have entered the stall of any horse with an infectious disease.

Most progressive farms use vaccinations to help manage disease. Deciding to use a specific vaccine for a recognized disease should be based on the risk the disease poses to those particular horses, the consequences of not vaccinating from both the economic and individual and herd health standpoint, and the possible adverse effects associated with the vaccination. In deciding which vaccines to use in the overall program, consider the age of the horses, their function, the number of animals and their density at the facility,

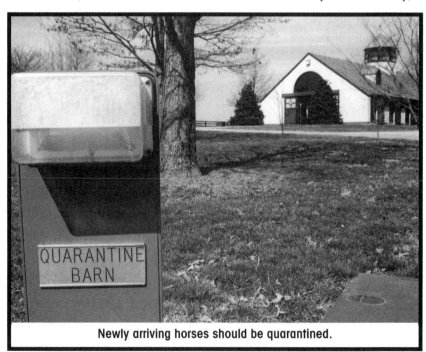

Newly arriving horses should be quarantined.

the cost of the program versus the benefits, the facility's management practices, and its location. Because many of these issues vary for individual animals and nearly all vary from farm to farm, there is no "standard" vaccination program for all horses or all facilities. Each situation must be evaluated independently. Owners or managers, with input from their veterinarian, should establish a vaccination program and prerequisites aimed at controlling the entry and spread of infectious disease.

Client expectations and the overall goals of a disease control program can vary significantly. Performance-horse management is centered on minimizing the time lost from training and competition. An animal that contracts an infectious disease usually requires time off. A horse's inability to compete and train can result in economic loss. However, the same disease in a backyard horse or a broodmare is unlikely to cause significant losses in money and time unless the horse is permanently impaired or the mare aborts.

CHAPTER 2

Principles of Vaccination

Vaccination plays a major part of a preventive medicine program, but many programs for individual horses and even for large stables are often based on incomplete understanding of the principles of vaccination and the particular needs of the animals for which the program is designed. For these reasons it is important to have realistic expectation based on a sound understanding of what particular vaccination programs provide.

Vaccination minimizes the risk of infection but does not prevent disease in all circumstances. To be effective, a primary series of vaccinations with a complete booster series must be administered prior to exposure to an infectious disease.

It should be noted, though, that not all horses respond similarly to a vaccine, and the duration of immunity against a particular infectious agent can vary. A herd approach to vaccination rather than an individual approach should be taken to control disease. This is extremely important in any barn in which diseases can be directly transmitted among horses. The time required to produce effective immunity from vaccination using a federally licensed vaccine is usually about two to three weeks after the primary series is completed, and one or more weeks after the routine booster is administered.

Presently, the efficacy of many of the commercially available equine vaccines is questionable. Indeed, few controlled studies have been conducted to evaluate their efficacy. Therefore, the use of vaccines should be considered only one component of the overall preventive medicine program aimed at limiting the incidence of disease. The other important components involve the use of all available information pertaining to various disease risk factors, modes of transmission, methods of early detection, appropriate quarantine of animals affected with contagious diseases, and good management practices aimed at preventing the transmission of disease by people or implements involved in the care of the affected horses. These have been outlined in the previous chapter.

AT A GLANCE

- Vaccination minimizes the risk of infection but does not prevent disease in all circumstances.

- Not all horses respond similarly to a vaccine, and the duration of immunity against a particular infectious agent can vary.

- A herd approach to vaccination should be taken to control disease rather than an individual approach.

The use of vaccines that are directed against more than one antigen, or multivalent vaccines, are common in many, if not most, equine practices. Despite their convenience, some very valid concerns should be considered. Use of multivalent vaccines presumes that there is one best time to vaccinate against all of the antigens contained within the vaccine. However, the periods of exposure to the disease-causing pathogens against which the vaccine is meant to protect may differ. Thus, the immunity produced and the height of protection may not occur when the risk of disease is greatest.

Secondly, the administration of multivalent vaccines also presumes that the same vaccine manufacturer produces the most effective vaccines against all of the diseases contained therein. Another major problem is that the duration of immunity for many of the vaccines contained within the multivalent vaccine is likely to be quite different. Therefore, administration of one multivalent vaccine twice a year may be adequate for coverage against one of the diseases, while immunity may have dissipated many months ago for another.

Finally, different horses are at different risk for various diseases. A "five-way" multivalent vaccine might contain one or more vaccines against a disease unlikely to be seen in an isolated horse or even on a small isolated farm. Meanwhile, the performance horse that is shipping frequently for competitions and encountering many other horses with unknown vaccination status from other areas is more likely to encounter less common diseases.

SIDE EFFECTS

Vaccination may be associated with a limited number of adverse effects. Muscle swelling, stiffness, mild fever, anorexia, and lethargy are all potential side effects. Systemic signs of malaise may be seen more commonly with the administration of intramuscular preparations of inactivated influenza virus vaccine than with others. This is thought to be due to reaction at the injection site. It is therefore recommended that horses do not receive any vaccination within two weeks of performance, sales, or shipment. It is further recommended that horses do not receive inactivated (killed) equine influenza vaccines within three weeks of international shipment. Other adverse reactions that have been associated with the administration of a vaccine include anaphylaxis and local irritation to the tissue, but these are uncommon. Anaphylaxis is a life-threatening emergency requiring immediate veterinary attention and possibly the administration of epinephrine, a cardiac drug that improves blood pressure while increasing heart rate and contractility. Local tissue reactions are generally self-limiting but may benefit from oral nonsteroidal anti-inflammatory drugs such as phenylbutazone or flunixin meglumine, warm compresses, topical DMSO gel, and gentle exercise. Local reactions might be minimized by vaccines deep in the semimembranosus and semitendinosus muscles of the hind leg and by allowing the horse to exercise after vaccination. Some horses appear to be sensitive to specific vaccines or vaccine types. Horses that react to multivalent vaccines might benefit from pre-medication with a nonsteroidal anti-inflammatory drug, administration of individual monovalent vaccines at different sites instead of using the multivalent vaccine, or from another brand of vaccine.

VACCINATING THE FOAL

The most important way of protecting a foal early in life against many common pathogens is to ensure adequate vaccination of the dam. Maternal antibodies are concentrated in the colostrum of the mare during the last trimester of gestation. Vaccination with a "full series" of vaccines is often advocated four to six weeks prior to foaling in order to maximize the levels of these antibodies within the colostrum. A good rule of thumb for the protection of the foal then is to vaccinate the mare appropriately for anything from which one wishes to protect the foal. The colostrum, or "first milk," is then highly concentrated with these antibodies when the foal nurses during the first 24 hours. During this time the foal's gastrointestinal tract is capable of absorbing these important antibodies. These antibodies then persist for six to nine months after foaling. However, the protective effects of these antibodies may begin to deteriorate well before this time — perhaps by two or three months of age. For this reason it has become popular to begin vaccinating these foals at or before this drop in protection.

Recent information indicates that the presence of even unprotective levels of maternally derived antibody may prevent an active immunologic response of the foal to vaccination. This maternal antibody may persist in the foal for six to nine months, depending on the antigen. Further, vaccination with killed equine influenza vaccine during the period of maternal antibody interference can blunt or retard the foal's immune response to vaccination, delaying the age at which the young horse is capable of producing appropriate immunity. Investigators recommend initial vaccination of the foal to begin after six months of age and perhaps as late as nine months. Effective vaccination in the face of maternally derived antibody will require the development of more potent vaccines that can effectively overcome interference from this antibody. As is the case for the administration of all first-time vaccines, a booster dose is required between three and six weeks after the original inoculation. Certain vaccines may require additional boosters. They will be mentioned when appropriate under their specific subheadings in the next chapter.

A specific mention of vaccination of foals for tetanus is warranted. With tetanus, as with any other pathogens, the most appropriate way to protect the foal is to ensure adequate colostrum intake following adequate vaccination of the mare and a booster two to six weeks prior to foaling. If such an approach is made and the level of antibodies in the foal is checked and found to be appropriate (IgG>800mg/dl), there is no need to administer either tetanus antitoxin or tetanus toxoid in the neonatal foal. In fact, it is unclear whether vaccination with tetanus toxoid at such an early stage confers immunity, does nothing, or is counterproductive. Administration of tetanus antitoxin to a foal out of a dam with an unknown vaccination history produces its effect for an unknown duration but is recommended. Tetanus antitoxin is not a vaccine. This means that it will bind circulating unbound toxin from the pathogen, *Clostridium tetani*, but once the antitoxin is eliminated or utilized, it has no residual protective effect. Overall then, the most effective and simplest way to protect the foal from tetanus is to vaccinate the mare appropriately and initiate tetanus vaccination in the foal between six and nine months of age.

DNA VACCINATION

DNA vaccination involves the induction of protein production by the introduction of DNA into cells in a way similar to natural infection with the antigen or organism against which the host is being vaccinated. This type of vaccination can produce both antibody production and cellular immune responses with no reported undesirable side effects. Such an approach may lead to the production of highly effective immunity in a safe and inexpensive manner. DNA vaccination has already proven to be useful in protecting horses from influenza virus, and there is some evidence of its effectiveness against equine herpesvirus. The development of such vaccines is only in the very early stages, but these vaccines appear to be promising.

CHAPTER 3

Individual Vaccines

INFLUENZA

Equine influenza is one of the most frequently encountered infectious diseases of horses. It affects the upper respiratory tract, producing illness associated with fever and coughing. There are numerous strains, and the occurrence of outbreaks may be associated with waning immunity of the equine population and emergence of a new strain. The risk of infection increases with horses that live in high-density and high-stress situations such as racetracks, training facilities, boarding stables, breeding farms, and show grounds. Equine influenza is introduced into a group of horses by a symptomatic or asymptomatic horse that is shedding the virus. The virus' highly contagious nature is facilitated through the spread of the pathogen by coughing or exposure to such objects as contaminated feed buckets or feeding equipment, grooming implements, or tack. The equine immune response is capable, however, of rapidly eliminating the virus. Infection can, therefore, be controlled or prevented from entering a horse population by strict quarantine of new horses for 14 days and by appropriate vaccination. Horses that are infected with an influenza virus shed the organism in the nasal secretions for up to 10 days.

Influenza is highly transmissible and is, therefore, important to consider in the vaccination program of any horse that regularly encounters new horses, is undergoing stressful situations in shipping and/or competitions, or is likely to encounter high-risk situations for disease transmission.

Today there are various manufacturers of equine influenza vaccines. Furthermore, both intramuscular (killed vaccines) and intranasal (modified live) vaccines are now available. The use of killed vaccines in the horse is associated with increases in circulating antibody in the vaccinated animal, but repeated vaccination with certain licensed vaccines of this type has failed to provide protection during outbreaks or reduce the severity of the disease. This may be related to the fact that these killed-virus vaccines cannot produce a local immune response at the level of infection (the respiratory system mucosa). Furthermore, the circulating antibody produced by the killed vaccines does not appear to be at high or persistent levels. However, these levels appear to be higher than those produced by the modified live vaccine (intranasal), and the killed vaccines are recommended for pregnant mares to facilitate the production of circulating antibody that is subsequently concentrated in the colostrum.

The levels of circulating antibody in the blood stream — even when there is a lot of it — do not necessarily mean the animal will be protected from the disease, suggesting that local responses in the upper respiratory tract may play an important role in the protection produced by this vaccine. Therefore, it seems that a major factor in the production of immunity by the intranasal vaccine is the production of the

AT A GLANCE

- Equine influenza, one of the most frequently encountered infectious diseases, is highly contagious.

- Tetanus is an extremely important vaccination to give all horses.

- Rabies is fatal and can be transmitted from horses to humans. All horses that are kept in or travel to areas where the virus is endemic should be vaccinated regularly.

- Conditionally licensed vaccines are now available for EPM and West Nile virus.

"local" or mucosal immune response — actually to prevent infection by not allowing the virus to enter the body. The circulating immunity produced cannot function unless the virus is already in the body, and then it is often not effective in preventing clinical signs. One currently licensed, modified live vaccine (FluAvert I. N., Heska Corp, Fort Collins, Colo.) has received significant support according to the results of published data. Field experience indicates that this vaccine is effective at preventing influenza.

Vaccination of foals with the killed vaccines in the presence of maternal antibody (derived from the colostrum) appears to induce a type of "immune-tolerance" during which foals and yearlings fail to respond to multiple doses administered over several months. For this reason it is important to initiate vaccination of foals after maternal antibody inhibition may be produced. Programs using the killed-virus vaccines (intramuscular) should therefore begin at nine months of age if the foals are isolated from new horses or horses that develop illness. This initial series should include three doses of vaccine administered at four- to six-week intervals. Foals that are born to unvaccinated mares may receive a primary vaccination series of three doses beginning at six months of age and at intervals of four to six weeks. The modified live-virus vaccine (intranasal) may be incorporated into the vaccination program instead of the killed (intramuscular) vaccine.

The modified live vaccine is recommended for administration to foals at 11 months of age. However, because it is unclear whether the maternal antibody interferes with the immune response to this vaccine, if vaccination of the foal with the modified live vaccine is performed before 11 months of age, it should be followed by a second dose when the foal is 11 months of age or older. Booster vaccination is recommended at six-month intervals and is not required before this as foals 11 months of age or older and previously unvaccinated adults appear to be protected after a single administration of the vaccine. Intranasal vaccination is particularly important when horses regularly commingle, in areas of frequent introduction of new animals, and for horses engaged in performance and showing. For programs that use the killed-virus vaccine (intramuscular), it is necessary to repeat vaccination in these horses at three- to four-month intervals in order to provide adequate circulating antibody levels in situations of high risk of exposure.

Because influenza outbreaks typically last three to four weeks and horses previously vaccinated or exposed to influenza are capable of mounting a rapid immune response, revaccination of healthy horses in the face of an outbreak is indeed beneficial in controlling the spread of disease. However, other control measures are also important, such as isolation of affected animals and appropriate management practices as previously described. The modified live vaccine is reported to be safe and highly effective in an outbreak, and may provide more rapid and complete immunity than the conventional killed vaccines.

RHINOPNEUMONITIS (HERPESVIRUS I AND IV)

Equine herpesviruses I and IV have been associated with several different types of disease in the horse. Equine herpesvirus IV is associated with respiratory disease, and equine herpesvirus I may cause three different manifestations of disease in the horse. Vaccination against herpesvirus infections is primarily indicated to prevent or reduce the incidence of viral abortion produced by EHV-I. A second manifestation of disease caused by EHV-I is central nervous system derangement or encephalomyelitis. The third form is respiratory disease. Horses infected with EHV-I and EHV-IV may become persistently and latently infected with the virus. Latently infected horses do not show clinical signs but may exhibit relapses of infection and viral shedding when stressed. Such characteristics of infection make the control of disease related to these viruses difficult. Although most mature horses do not manifest clinical respiratory disease with EHV-I or EHV-IV infections, they also do not appear to develop resistance to the abortogenic or neurologic forms of EHV-I infection, even with repeated exposure.

Though EHV-I and EHV-IV infect susceptible animals via the respiratory tract through nasal secretions of affected horses by both direct and indirect contact, little information conclusively indicates these viruses to be significant respiratory tract pathogens in horses of any age. Surveillance studies involving performance horses have also failed to clearly associate EHV-I and EHV-IV with outbreaks of respiratory disease. However, EHV-I as a cause of abortion in pregnant mares poses significant threat to other pregnant mares by spread from and contact with aborted fetuses, fetal fluids, and placentas. For this reason, management practices are very important in controlling the spread of this manifestation of the disease. Appropriate handling and disposal of fetal tissues from an abortion are imperative. It is also important to have the fetus and placenta appropriately handled and examined by a veterinarian and a pathologist in order to identify EHV-I-related abortions due to the implications that such abortion carries for other pregnant mares from the same farm.

To date, only two vaccines are labeled for use and prevention of abortion in mares (Pneumabort K®+ 1b and Prodigy®). These vaccines are monovalent and killed-virus preparations. Clinically, consistent use of these vaccines appears to reduce the incidence of abortion storms, but sporadic abortion and "outbreaks" of abortion have been reported in vaccinated animals. It is recommended that pregnant mares be vaccinated with one of the monovalent vaccines labeled for prevention of abortion at five, seven, and nine months of gestation. Some veterinarians advocate administration of the vaccine beginning at three months of gestation; still others administer the vaccine at four, six, eight, and 10 months of gestation so that the entire booster series can be given to the pregnant mare at four weeks before foaling (for colostral antibody production). Another approach involves the administration of a bivalent killed vaccine against both EHV-I and EHV-IV at the time of breeding, and again at four to six weeks before foaling in order to maximize colostral antibody against these pathogens. Such vaccination, however, does not preclude pregnant mares from needing the monovalent vaccines that are labeled to prevent abortion. It is recommended to vaccinate barren mares and stallions prior to breeding season and then at six-month intervals in order to reduce viral shedding and potential infection of pregnant mares.

Both the killed bivalent EHV-I/EHV-IV vaccines and the modified live EHV-I and -IV vaccines have been used in programs aimed at preventing respiratory disease in foals, weanlings, yearlings, and young horses in performance events of all types. Using these vaccines in an effort to prevent respiratory disease is questionable for several reasons. It remains unclear what role, if any, EHV-I and EHV-IV play in the development of clinical respiratory disease. And there is a general lack of information supporting the efficacy of these vaccines in the prevention of infection with these viruses.

Maternal antibody interference has been shown to block the serologic response of most foals to vaccination with the killed bivalent preparations of EHV-I/EHV-IV until the foals are past five months of age. Three or more doses of such killed vaccines are necessary to produce protective immunity. If vaccination is initiated at the appropriate time when maternal antibody interference is less likely (after six months), the foals will be seven to eight months of age before protective immunity would be present. It then becomes difficult to explain how these vaccines would be useful in the prevention of respiratory disease commonly associated with EHV infections since they are reported to be most common around the time of weaning. The modified live preparation of EHV-I (Rhinomune®) has been shown to produce cellular immunity in foals despite the presence of maternal antibody, but whether such immunity protects against natural infection is unclear.

Although the role of EHV-I and EHV-IV as respiratory pathogens is unclear, many practitioners vaccinate against EHV-I and EHV-IV regularly. Primary vaccination of foals usually begins with the administration of three doses of the live or killed EHV-I/EHV-IV vaccine beginning at four to six months of age and at three- to six-week intervals thereafter. Weanlings, yearlings, and young performance horses at high risk of exposure are revaccinated at three- to six-month intervals. For mature horses, revaccination of nonpregnant animals is not necessary unless they reside on breeding farms. Again, this method of vaccination remains questionable. Vaccination against EHV-I is ineffective in preventing the neurologic form of disease.

EASTERN/WESTERN/VENEZUELAN EQUINE ENCEPHALOMYELITIS

These diseases are caused by viruses that infect birds, small mammals, and reptiles. Such animals serve as a natural reservoir for these viruses, and the risk of equine exposure appears to be related to the season and the distribution of insect vectors capable of transmitting the viruses to horses. Transmission of the viruses between these intermediate hosts and horses probably occurs through blood-sucking insects such as mosquitoes. Infections with WEE occur predominantly in the western United States, western Canada, and South America. Sporadic cases of WEE have been reported in the northeast and southeast regions of the United States. The distribution of EEE appears to be primarily in the eastern and southeastern United States, the West Indies, Central America, and South America. VEE is restricted to Central America and South America and the West Indies. VEE is considered to be an exotic disease to the United States.

However, outbreaks have been recorded in the United States. It is recommended that all horses in this country be vaccinated against Eastern and Western equine encephalomyelitis. Further, horses that reside in or are traveling to areas where the risk of exposure to Venezuelan equine encephalomyelitis is increased should be vaccinated. At-risk horses might be traveling to or competing in areas of the country neighboring Central America, particularly along the Mexican border.

Vaccination against one of these viruses does not confer protection against all of them. Vaccinations should be administered to horses prior to the mosquito season. The duration of immunity is about six months for horses vaccinated with inactivated bivalent (EEE/WEE) or trivalent (EEE/WEE/VEE) preparations. For horses in areas where the mosquito season is longer than six months or for horses that are competing in areas where some of these viruses are endemic, vaccinate every four to six months to maximize continual protection.

Vaccination of foals should begin at six months of age if the mare was vaccinated against these viruses four to six weeks prior to foaling and the foal subsequently received adequate colostral antibody. Colostral antibody appears to protect the foal for up to six or seven months of age. The primary series of vaccination involves three doses administered at three- to six-week intervals and revaccination at one year of age. Vaccination of foals born to unvaccinated mares can begin at three to four months of age. In such cases, the initial vaccination series follows the same schedule: three doses of vaccine at three- to six-week intervals with a booster vaccination at one year of age. Foals born in particularly high-risk areas should begin the outlined primary vaccination series at three to four months of age. Vaccination should be repeated every six months in situations of continual or repetitive exposure to mosquitoes, or two to four weeks prior to exposure to mosquitoes or to mosquito season. Revaccination against these diseases is frequently coupled with tetanus immunization using multivalent vaccines.

The viral encephalidites are theoretically transmissible to humans in whom they cause encephalitis similar to that seen in the equine species. However, horse-to-human transmission has not been documented, probably due to the relatively brief period the virus is circulating in the horse. However, the possible risk to humans may be another reason to consider vaccination of all horses against these diseases.

TETANUS

Tetanus is an extremely important vaccination to give any and all horses, as the organism *Clostridium tetani* is a primary soil contaminant and is found throughout the environment and in the intestinal tract and feces of horses, as well as of other animals and human beings. The organism produces a toxin that can cause spastic paralysis leading to death; horses are particularly susceptible to the toxin's effects. The disease is expensive to treat and has a high mortality rate. The organism typically enters through a wound, contaminating it, and the subsequent development of an oxygen-free environment allows the production of the toxin. The toxin causes spastic paralysis by inhibiting central nervous system cells that control muscle spasm. Because of horses' great sensitivity to it and because tetanus-causing bacteria may be present in many types of soils, all horses should be vaccinated for this disease.

Tetanus toxoid vaccination is believed to be highly effective and should be boosted annually as well as when a tetanus-prone lesion is sustained. Manufacturers of the toxoid recommend initiating immunization with a primary series of two doses given three to eight weeks apart and annual boosters thereafter. In North America tetanus has been reported in vaccinated horses; therefore, vaccination intervals longer than one year are not advised. Vaccinated horses that sustain a wound or undergo surgery more than six months after the last tetanus immunization should receive a booster with tetanus toxoid.

Pregnant mares should be vaccinated four to six weeks before foaling, for both the mare's benefit and for the concentration of specific immunoglobulins in the colostrum. Maternal antibodies that are passively transferred to the foal in the colostrum are reported to interfere significantly with the foal's ability to mount an immune response to vaccination with the toxoid until about six months of age. Foals receiving adequate transfer of maternally derived antibody from mares that were appropriately vaccinated prior to foaling should, therefore, be given an initial tetanus toxoid vaccine at six months of age followed by the completion of the primary series by revaccination twice at four- to six-week intervals. Foals born to unvaccinated dams require the initial series to begin at three to four months of age. Three doses of toxoid are recommended in the primary series for all foals because it appears that a significant proportion of foals do not seroconvert (produce antibody) after a two-dose series regardless of whether maternal antibodies are present. Foals born to unvaccinated dams are recommended to have 1,500 units of tetanus antitoxin at the time of birth.

Tetanus antitoxin should be considered in unvaccinated horses that have sustained a wound or undergone surgery. Immediate protection conferred by the antitoxin lasts approximately three weeks with a dose of 1,500 units. A small number of horses may develop serum hepatitis and liver failure related to the administration of tetanus antitoxin several weeks after administration. This condition can be fatal. Therefore, it is preferable to maintain adequate immunization using the toxoid rather than having to give antitoxin to an unvaccinated horse.

The unvaccinated horse should concurrently receive a tetanus toxoid vaccine at the time of injury or surgery, administered from a separate syringe. It is important to recall that these horses will still require a second and third dose of the toxoid at four- to eight-week intervals to complete the primary series. Annual boosters will be necessary thereafter.

BOTULISM

Botulism is a disease caused by a toxin produced by the bacterium *Clostridium botulinum*. As in the case of tetanus, toxin is produced by a clostridial organism. However, instead of the spastic paralysis produced by tetanus, botulism produces flaccid paralysis and weakness when nerve transmission to the muscle is inhibited by the binding of toxin and blockage of nerve-to-muscle transmission. Botulism is the most potent biologic toxin known, and horses are highly sensitive to its presence and effects. The clinical effect on the horse may become severe enough to cause the horse to become recumbent and eventually to die from paralysis of respiratory muscles.

There are three major forms of botulism, which are categorized by the mode of entry of the toxin. Ingestion of pre-formed endotoxin (forage poisoning) from contaminated feedstuffs may be the most common means of entry. Ingestion of the *Clostridium botulinum* spores may lead to production of toxin within the gastrointestinal tract, as is most commonly the mechanism in foals (shaker foal syndrome). These types of botulism may be associated with contaminated feed or hay and may be a particular concern for horses being fed round bales or grazing in pastures with animal carcasses or decaying plant material. Finally, infection of a wound with *Clostridium botulinum* may lead to the production of the toxin after the spores vegetate.

There are eight recognized types of botulism toxin. Horses appear to be most susceptible to types B and C. Almost all cases of shaker foal syndrome appear to be caused by type B toxin, and foals between two weeks and seven months of age in Kentucky and Mid-Atlantic seaboard states appear to be at greatest risk. However, shaker foal syndrome is reported spo-radically in other areas of the country.

There appears to be a geographic distribution of the sub-types. Type A appears to be concentrated in areas west of the Rocky Mountains, type B in Kentucky and in the Mid-Atlantic seaboard, and type C found more commonly in Florida. To date, the available toxoid vaccine (BotTox-B) is directed only against type B toxin, and there is no cross-protection provid-ed to other types of botulism toxin. Therefore, in addition to vaccination, methods for the control of botulism should involve good husbandry: vermin removal, disposal of animal carcasses, and avoidance of spoiled feedstuffs.

Vaccination of pregnant mares produces protection in the foal against type B botulism (shaker foal syndrome) but should be restricted to the final trimester of pregnancy. Pregnant mares that have not been previously vaccinated should receive a primary series of three doses adminis-tered four weeks apart and scheduled so that the final dose is administered four to six weeks before foaling. Mares that have already received the initial series can be boosted at four to six weeks prior to foaling in order to maximize pro-tection conferred by colostral antibody to the foal. Maternal antibody in the foal does not appear to inhibit the development of an immune response and production of antibody by the foal itself; thus, vaccination of the foal can begin at two to three months of age or older in endemic areas. The primary series in the foal should consist of three doses administered at four-week intervals. All other horses should also receive a three-dose primary series at four-week intervals and a yearly booster vaccination thereafter. For broodmares, yearly boosters are best timed at four to six weeks before foaling.

Horses that develop clinical disease associated with botu-lism toxin may be treated with intravenously administered botulism antitoxin. However, the administration of the anti-toxin carries no effect for toxin that is already bound to receptors in the junction between the nerve and muscle. The utility of the antitoxin is in its ability to bind toxin that is still circulating. Clinical signs of the horse may continue to deteriorate for 24 hours beyond the administration of the toxin. Recovery of the horse is optimal when the animal has received antitoxin, the progression of clinical signs is slow, and the horse does not become recumbent. The recommended dose of the type B antitoxin is 30,000 IU for the foal and 70,000 IU for an adult horse.

POTOMAC HORSE FEVER

This disease is caused by an organism called *Ehrlichia risticii* and is known as equine monocytic erhlichiosis. Clinical syndromes produced by this organism may include equine ehrlichial colitis and/or equine ehrlichial abortion. Although the common manifestation of colitis in horses is profuse, watery diarrhea, true diarrhea may occur in less than 60 percent of cases of Potomac Horse Fever. Clinical signs may, therefore, include colic, biphasic fever, anorexia, and laminitis. Abortion induced by this organism is often seen after the mare has recovered from equine ehrlichial colitis and may occur late in gestation. Placentitis and a retained placenta often accompany abortion, and the organism may be identified by examination of the fetal colon.

The disease caused by *Ehrlichia risticii* got its name from the original description of the disease in horses from the northeastern and Mid-Atlantic regions near the Potomac River. However, since that time, the disease has been described in other regions of the United States and Canada. The disease tends to occur sporadically and does not appear to be directly transmitted from horse to horse. It appears that accidental ingestion of aquatic insects that harbor a certain life stage of snails that are infected with the ehrlichial organism is one possible mode of transmission. Evidence indicates that the incidence of disease fluctuates, with the highest number of cases being reported in July, August, and September. Foals appear to be at a lower risk for the disease. Natural infection with the organism appears to produce a strong antibody response and duration of immunity lasting 20 months or longer.

The available vaccinations against Potomac Horse Fever are labeled for the aid of prevention of the disease caused by the ehrlichial organism. The efficacy of the vaccine in the prevention of disease has not been established, and the vaccine may be most useful in reducing the severity of clinical disease, according to some veterinarians who practice in areas where the disease is endemic. Experimental studies have suggested the provision of at least partial protection of limited duration.

Horses that might benefit most from vaccination include those residing within endemic areas, those living on farms that have had another animal affected by this disease, and those traveling to areas where the disease has been recognized. The recommended vaccination protocol is initiated with a primary series of two doses three to four weeks apart for adult horses that have not been previously vaccinated. Revaccination is recommended by the manufacturer at six-to-12-month intervals, but at six months after vaccination, only about 50 percent of horses appear to be protected. Therefore, a shorter vaccination interval with revaccination at four-month intervals has been recommended for continuous protection.

Because the disease appears to have a seasonal occurrence, revaccination has also been practiced in the late spring just before the first cases might be expected, followed by a second vaccination in four months to maximize protection during the period of greatest disease risk. Vaccination of the foal begins at five or six months of age due to the low incidence of disease in foals and the possibility of maternal antibody interference. Pregnant mares vaccinated four to six weeks prior to foaling will concentrate and transfer antibody against the organism through the colostrum. Foals that receive the primary series of vaccination before five months of age should get a three-dose primary series at four-week intervals, rather than the two-dose series recommended by the manufacturer.

STRANGLES

Strangles is caused by the bacterium *Streptococcus equi var. equi* and affects the upper respiratory system of the horse. The disease primarily affects younger horses such as weanlings and yearlings, but horses of any age can be affected. The disease often causes thick nasal discharge with fever and lymph node swelling that often progresses to abscessation of the lymph nodes. Lymph nodes may break open and drain pus, laden with bacteria and capable of causing disease in other horses. Nasal discharge from affected horses is also infectious. The nature of the organism and its mode of transmission make this disease highly contagious among susceptible horses. Direct contact with infected horses and indirect transmission by contaminated water troughs, feed bunks, pastures, stalls, trailers, tack, and grooming equipment may lead to transmission of the organism to other susceptible horses. Horses that have had clinical disease due to strangles may shed the organism for weeks to months after clinical recovery (average time about six weeks). Following natural infection with the organism, most horses (about 70 percent) develop long-term immunity to reinfection, whereas a smaller percentage (30 percent) develop immunity that lasts for a few months.

There are two types of vaccines now available for the prevention of strangles. One is directed at a particular subunit of the bacterium called the M-protein. These inactivated vaccines (StrepVax II® and Strepgard®) are administered intramuscularly. Although these vaccines do not lead to the production of antibody capable of preventing infection, there is significant evidence that the systemic antibody produced is effective in reducing the severity and duration of clinical signs of infection and the overall incidence of disease in outbreak situations. Despite these findings, the M-protein subunit vaccines should not be expected universally to prevent infection and the development of strangles. The second type of vaccine now available is a modified live vaccine for administration by intranasal route (Pinnacle I.N.®). Its efficacy appears to be improved over that of the M-protein subunit vaccines, but it too does not necessarily provide universal protection against the development of disease.

Vaccination against *Streptococcous equi var. equi* is not routinely recommended except in situations in which the cost of not vaccinating outweighs the cost of vaccination. Such instances occur when strangles is a persistent problem on the premises and/or the occurrence of strangles in the horse herd may be associated with significant loss of value of the animal (such as in young horses being prepared for sale). Unless an outbreak occurs, vaccination is not routinely recommended for pleasure or performance horses, as these animals are generally exposed to low-risk situations.

Use of the M-protein subunit vaccines requires a series of two or three doses in the primary vaccination series beginning at four to six months of age and given at three- to six-week intervals. Annual vaccination is recommended thereafter, but efficacy appears to improve with an initial three-dose series and revaccination at six-month intervals. On breeding farms where there is high risk of strangles epidemics, foals are initially protected by vaccinating pregnant mares four to six weeks prior to foaling with an M-protein subunit vaccine to enhance colostral immunoglobulin concentrations passed to the foals. The modified live vaccine (Pinnacle I. N.®) is preferable to the inactivated M-protein vaccines for primary vaccination of high-risk foals and adult horses.

The initial vaccination series using this product should begin at four to six months of age using a series of two doses that are administered at intervals of two to three weeks. It is recommended that a third dose then be administered three months later and boosters be given yearly or every six months for higher risk situations. If the intranasal vaccine is administered to foals less than two months of age, administration of another dose of vaccine (modified live) is recommended between two and four weeks prior to weaning, a high-risk period. However, foals are unlikely to benefit from vaccination with the intranasal vaccine prior to four months of age due to the inability to manufacture antibody associated with the response to intranasal vaccines at that age. It also is unknown whether maternal antibody inhibition occurs with this vaccine.

Outbreaks of strangles tend to be persistent on breeding farms and may last for months to well over a year. Strangles vaccination is a worthwhile consideration in an outbreak to help control the spread of disease to susceptible animals. However, whenever strangles is recognized, prompt and strict isolation of all affected horses should be instituted to help control spread of disease. Vaccination of horses that have not been exposed to any affected horses or contaminated materials may be helpful but not sufficient to control the highly contagious nature of the organism and the outbreak. It appears that the modified live vaccine (intranasal) is both safe and effective for use in an outbreak and may produce an immune response more rapidly in previously unvaccinated horses. Horses that have been vaccinated can generate an effective immune response more rapidly than those that have not. The intranasal vaccine is reported to be safe in pregnant mares and may also be used in these animals in the face of an outbreak.

The injectable M-protein subunit vaccines are associated with relatively common local reactions at the injection site. Such reactions are most frequently mild and cause muscle pain at the injection site. Less commonly, there may be signs of fever, depression, anorexia, and abscessation at the injection site. Purpura hemorrhagica is a rare complication of all strangles vaccines. This condition is produced when there is an immune-mediated reaction that results in swelling of the limbs and/or hemorrhages on the surfaces of mucous membranes. This complication can become life-threatening, underscoring the need to restrict the administration of these vaccines by a licensed veterinarian. The modified live vaccine (intranasal) can cause injection site abscesses if it is inadvertently administered intramuscularly by the contamination of needles used to administer other vaccines or other medications. For this reason, it is recommended that all injectables (vaccines and others) be administered to the horse before handling and administering the modified live (intranasal) vaccine. Some other reported adverse responses to the intranasal vaccine include nasal discharge, lymph node swelling, lymph node abscessation, limb swelling, and, rarely, internal abscessation.

RABIES

A virus that persists in wildlife in infected animals causes rabies. It can be transmitted to the horse through a bite wound from an infected animal. The disease causes central nervous system derangement and is fatal. Also, because the disease is transmissible to humans from horses, vaccination should be mandatory in areas where the virus is known to exist in wildlife. The wildlife species that serve as a reservoir for the virus differ from region to region throughout the country. All horses that are kept or travel to areas where the virus is endemic should be vaccinated regularly. There are a number of vaccines now available that are licensed for use in the horse. The dosage quantity usually administered is 2cc, rather than 1cc, which is given to small animals. The vaccines used are killed-virus preparations. Modified live-virus preparations not licensed for use in horses should not be used.

The initial vaccination series involves the administration of three doses of vaccine three to six weeks apart in previously unvaccinated adult horses. Primary vaccination in the foals of unvaccinated mares should begin at three months of age or older. The first dose is then followed by a second dose at one year of age and yearly vaccination thereafter. Maternally derived antibody from colostrum ingestion by the foal does appear to interfere with immunization of foals. Therefore, foals born to vaccinated mares should receive their first dose of rabies vaccine at no earlier than six months of age; the second dose is administered four weeks later, and the third dose is given at one year of age. Annual revaccination is necessary thereafter. None of the vaccines labeled for use in horses is labeled for use in pregnant mares; however, some veterinarians do administer the killed virus vaccine to pregnant mares without problem. Otherwise, it is necessary to vaccinate mares prior to breeding.

EQUINE VIRAL ARTERITIS

Equine viral arteritis is a contagious disease caused by the equine arteritis virus, which is found throughout the world. The disease produced by the virus may be very similar to that which is caused by respiratory viruses and varies in severity of clinical signs. Other commonly associated clinical signs of disease caused by this virus might include fever, decreased appetite, swelling of the limbs and other generalized areas of the body, tearing, nasal discharge, skin rashes, pneumonia, and death of young foals. Pregnant mares may abort in response to infection with the virus. A long-term carrier state can follow infection in stallions during which the virus can be shed in the semen. All breeds appear to be susceptible to infection with the equine arteritis virus; however, seroprevalence indicates that seroconversion and infection may be particularly high in Standardbreds. Standardbreds often have antibody against the virus but seldom are affected with the clinical disease — they may harbor the virus but have a more effective immune response that controls the expression of the clinical signs. Although a major route of transmission is by inhalation of aerosolized nasal secretions from horses with clinical disease, of greater importance may be the transmission of the virus to mares from chronically infected stallions through semen by natural or artificial breeding.

A modified live-virus vaccine (Arvac®) was developed and used successfully to control an outbreak that occurred in Kentucky in 1984. The vaccine was shown to be safe and useful during this outbreak. The vaccine is used in horses to prevent infection and the induction of the long-term carrier state in stallions and to protect non-pregnant mares that are being bred to stallions that carry and may shed the virus. The vaccination has been used to control outbreaks of EVA at racetracks.

Vaccination with a single dose in unvaccinated horses appears to be sufficient to produce protective immunity without requiring repeat doses. Annual boosters appear sufficient thereafter. Strategic use of the vaccine has been a major component in the control of EVA in the Kentucky Thoroughbred population. Appropriate use of the vaccine is facilitated by consultation with state control veterinarians.

Vaccination of breeding stallions is performed yearly about one month prior to the breeding season in order to prevent establishment of the carrier state. Young pre-pubertal colts and breeding stallions should receive serum antibody testing before the initial vaccination to screen for potential carriers. After vaccination with the modified live vaccine, seroconversion will occur, and, therefore, using serology as a screening test for carrier state becomes useless. Mares to be bred to carrier stallions will need to be vaccinated at least three weeks before breeding to prevent fetal loss and infection of the mare. Vaccinated mares will shed the virus after being bred, and, therefore, should be isolated for three weeks. The vaccine is not recommended for use in pregnant mares, particularly in the last two months of gestation. Foaling mares should be vaccinated after foaling and before being rebred. Foals less than six weeks of age should not be vaccinated unless the risk of exposure to the virus is high.

Foals born to seropositive mares become seropositive themselves after ingesting colostrum. Maternally derived antibody is present in the foal until about seven months of age. Vaccination of the foal at eight months of age or older is, therefore, adequate to minimize the likelihood of maternal antibody interference. Breeds in which the virus is particularly prevalent should have the intact males between eight and 12 months of age vaccinated to prevent them from becoming carriers. The seroconversion of vaccinated horses may present a complication for horses that are to be exported because the antibody present after seroconversion is present after natural exposure to the virus as well as after vaccination. Therefore, it is impossible to differentiate the vaccinated horse from the horse that was exposed to and/or that carries the virus.

ROTAVIRUS

Equine rotavirus is an infectious cause of diarrhea in foals during the first few weeks of life. Outbreaks of diarrhea may occur with the virus on farms with young foals. Older foals and adult horses appear to develop resistance to infection and to diarrhea due to the virus. The virus is associated with damage to the small intestine with associated malabsorption and maldigestion. There are a number of serogroups, serotypes, and genotypes recognized; however, the commonly identified types are of the A serogroup, the G3 serotype, and the P12 genotype. Other isolates of rotavirus are untyped, and it remains possible that these other isolates may differ in serogroup and serotype and/or genotype and may be associated with the generation of clinical disease in young foals.

A killed rotavirus A (serogroup) vaccine has been produced against the G3 serotype and is conditionally licensed for use in this country. It is recommended for administration to pregnant mares in endemic areas as an aid in the prevention of rotavirus A-induced diarrhea in foals. A three-dose series is required at eight, nine, and 10 months of pregnancy. When used accordingly, the vaccine is reported to increase serum antibody levels in the mare and thereby the concentration of the antibody in her colostrum. Passive transfer of the antibody by ingestion of colostrum by the foal produces increased antibody levels in foals that were born to and have suckled from vaccinated mares.

Field studies have indicated the vaccine to be safe and at least partially protective. However, some veterinarians believe the vaccine to be marginally effective in preventing the disease and that it may reduce severity of clinical signs of the disease in the foal at best. This could indicate that the prevention of infection and disease caused by rotavirus requires a different type of immunity, such as intestinal mucosal immunity. This type of immunity does not appear to be significantly induced by this vaccine. Therefore, complete protection from rotaviral diarrhea is unlikely to be produced by the administration of this vaccine. Furthermore, this vaccine does not protect against disease that may be produced by other strains of the virus.

ANTHRAX

With today's increased concern for bioterrorism, it is likely that veterinarians and their clients will discuss vaccination against anthrax. Anthrax is a disease caused by a spore-forming bacterium, *Bacillus anthracis*. The disease is serious and can be rapidly fatal to both animals and human beings. In humans there are generally three forms of the disease: cutaneous (skin) anthrax, intestinal anthrax, and respiratory anthrax. Transmission to animals and humans occurs with ingestion, inhalation, or contamination of wounds by soil-borne spores from areas where soil alkalinity permits survival of the organism or from animals that have died from the disease.

A live spore vaccine (anthrax spore vaccine) has been used to vaccinate horses at risk of exposure to the organism. A primary series of two doses is recommended to be administered two to three weeks apart and annual booster vaccination thereafter. Clinical evidence supports the presumption of protection conferred by this vaccine, but vaccination of pregnant mares is not advised. The use of antibiotics at the time of administration of this vaccine, particularly those that are effective against *Bacillus anthracis*, must be avoided in order to prevent inadequate response to vaccination using this live spore vaccine. Both local injection site and systemic adverse reactions have been reported with use of this vaccine.

EQUINE PROTOZOAL MYELOENCEPHALITIS (EPM)

EPM is a disease caused by a protozoan parasite. It affects the central nervous system of a very small percentage of horses that are exposed to the parasite. Recently, a killed vaccine has been produced and labeled for vaccination of healthy horses as an aid in the prevention of neurologic disease (equine protozoal myeloencephalitis) caused by subsequent exposure to the protozoan *Sarcocystis neurona*. The clinical disease of EPM manifests in a number of ways, but the typical presentation involves mild to severe gait deficits. Affected horses may show signs of incoordination, stumbling, unsteadiness, and less common signs such as severe muscle atrophy, cranial nerve deficits, and seizures. The clinical signs depend on the areas of the central nervous system that are affected and may mimic any disease that affects the equine central nervous system and some forms of musculoskeletal disease and lameness.

The USDA has issued a conditional license for an EPM vaccine. Such a license means that the vaccine has been shown to be safe, pure, and to have a reasonable expectation of efficacy in preventing illness. The vaccine is shown to stimulate the development of neutralizing antibodies to *Sarcocystis neurona*, but it is yet unclear whether these antibodies are capable of providing adequate protection to prevent infection and/or clinical disease. Horses exposed naturally to *Sarcocystis neurona* and vaccinated horses have similar circulating antibodies. This antibody has formed the basis of blood and CSF testing. However, the naturally occurring antibodies have not been effective in preventing disease. The efficacy of this vaccine is therefore undefined.

Reliable testing of the vaccine's efficacy may be delayed, since it is difficult to induce the disease in horses experimentally. However, numerous vaccines are on the market for which efficacy trials have not been conducted but that may play a role in reducing the severity and/or the rate of occurrence of the disease. Use of this vaccine should be thoroughly discussed with a qualified veterinarian, weighing the benefits of vaccination against the costs, likelihood of exposure to the organism, likelihood of development of the disease after exposure, and the results of field experience or trials pertaining to the vaccine's efficacy.

Vaccination is likely to complicate diagnosis of EPM further, since horses that may have tested negative for antibody against the organism in the serum and cerebrospinal fluid will convert to positive after receiving the vaccine. The recommended vaccination schedule has not yet been determined. At this time, Ft. Dodge recommends an initial series of two doses, with three to six weeks between these injections. Because the vaccine is a killed preparation, the immune response might be improved by administering a third dose again in another three to six weeks after the second dose. Annual revaccination is recommended thereafter.

WEST NILE VIRUS

West Nile Virus was first recognized in 1999 when outbreaks occurred in the northeastern United States. The virus affects humans and horses as incidental hosts of the virus, which circulates among wild birds by transmission through insect vectors such as mosquitoes. Horses appear to be affected by the virus more commonly than other domestic animals. The clinical signs relate to the development of encephalitis or inflammation of the brain. Many horses that become infected do not develop illness, but in 1999 and 2000 about 38 percent of those that were clinically affected did not survive.

Control of the disease should focus on the control of mosquito populations and the rate of exposure of horses to mosquitoes. Reduction of mosquito breeding sites involves disposing of any water-holding containers and all other potential sources of stagnant water because mosquitoes can breed in any small puddle that lasts for longer than four days. Screened housing, properly used insect repellents such as synthetic pyrethroid compounds (e.g., permethrin), and keeping horses stabled at night may help reduce exposure to mosquitoes.

In addition to these management measures, a conditionally licensed vaccine is now available for use in horses. The vaccine has met the requirements for this license by showing safety, purity, and a reasonable expectation of efficacy in preventing illness. The product is a killed-virus preparation, which the manufacturer recommends be given in two doses three to six weeks apart. As is the case for killed vaccines in general, there may be benefit to the administration of a third dose three to six weeks after the second dose.

There is no specific information regarding booster vaccination. As the disease and characteristics of this virus are likely to be similar to the diseases and viruses causing EEE, WEE, and VEE, it may be necessary to booster vaccination at six-month intervals for continuous protection. However, this is unclear as yet, and yearly vaccination may be all that is required. Because the virus is transmitted by mosquitoes in similar fashion to the other viral encephalidites, vaccination might also be advised prior to mosquito season and/or prior to traveling to areas where this season is prolonged.

CHAPTER 4

Principles of Deworming

P arasite control programs should be designed to reduce infections and diseases caused by parasites and to minimize transmission of parasites among horses. Infestation with gastrointestinal parasites reduces the benefits of feed and nutrients and increases incidence of colic and loose manure or diarrhea. Larval migration of gastrointestinal parasites can be associated with other clinical diseases such as parasitic pneumonia and neurologic disorders. Other parasites, such as some external parasites, may cause hypersensitivity reactions in the skin and development of wounds in certain areas.

A thorough parasite control program involves a complete understanding of helpful management practices and knowing how different types of dewormers work. Because management practices, economics, location, and disease outbreaks differ, no one program for parasite control applies universally. A veterinarian should help customize an individual program for each farm or situation. Today's programs might include interval deworming (fast, slow, and no rotation), daily deworming, strategic deworming, and targeted deworming. All have advantages and disadvantages. The success, selection, and need to modify a deworming program are generally dictated by the degree of control of the cyathostome parasites (small strongyles) and their encysted stages within the individual horse and/or the population of horses. A program that includes "tube deworming" is no longer necessary and probably offers no real advantage other than assuring the complete delivery of the dewormer to the stomach. The risk of overdosing the horse by overestimating weight is reduced by the safety margins of today's dewormers. Furthermore, an experienced horseman is able to administer paste dewormers effectively without significant loss of the medication. Horses that are to receive a paste of any kind should have all hay and feed removed from the mouth to prevent loss of the medication with the dropping of the feedstuff.

FAST ROTATION INTERVAL DEWORMING

Fast rotation interval deworming alternates different classes of dewormers during the year at predetermined periods (usually four to six weeks). It increases intervals between treatments with the same class of drug and thus reduces development of resistance. This allows elimination of parasites not uniformly killed by all drugs (*Gasterophilus spp.*, *Anoplocephala perfoliata*/*A. magna*). A disadvantage is that the egg reappearance period for different drugs is variable (ivermectin, eight to 10 weeks; other drugs, four to six weeks). Therefore, using standard intervals between treatments with different drug classes may not minimize pasture contamination. Despite this, some exposure to parasites in this way may actually help by allowing some protective immunity to develop. A fast rotation interval deworming program will likely cost more than most deworming programs. As with all deworming programs, well-timed administration of ivermectin or moxidectin to eliminate stomach bots and administration of 2-3x pyrantel to eliminate tapeworms is necessary. Treat with ivermectin in late spring (May) and fall (November) for elimination of bots. Yearly deworming with a double dose of fenbendazole for five consecutive days to control encysted small strongyles may be appropriate despite the apparent broad spectrum of control offered by the fast rotation interval deworming program.

ANNUAL (SLOW) ROTATION

Slow or annual rotation uses the same anthelmintic or class of anthelmintic at appropriate intervals throughout the year. The drug classes are alternated yearly rather than with every dosing. This approach does not account for the varying effectiveness of dewormers against a broad range of parasites but particularly focuses on treatment and control of cyathostomes. Therefore, it is important to administer other dewormers such as ivermectin and pyrantel to eliminate parasites not killed by the drug being used that year. Timely administrations of ivermectin and 2-3x pyrantel will be necessary to bolster the program to address stomach bots and tapeworms. Larvicidal doses (double doses) of fenbendazole for five consecutive days also may be appropriate.

NO ROTATION

Programs that use no rotation involve the continued use of one effective drug until it no longer reduces small strongyle numbers as indicated by fecal egg counts. The intervals of administration depend on the dewormer used, but this program is limited to the use of ivermectin or the daily administration of pyrantel tartrate (Strongid® C).

One benefit is that such a program is easily implemented and provides maximal reduction of parasite burdens. Rapid resistance has not been seen to develop with such programs. Horses raised on no-rotation programs will acquire resistance more slowly. The administration of 2-3x pyrantel to control tapeworms would be necessary with either the use of ivermectin or pyrantel as the anthelmintic. This is necessary even with the use of pyrantel tartrate, as the daily dosage is well below the required 2-3x dosage. If pyrantel tartrate is used, ivermectin would be necessary at the appropriate times (May and November) to control stomach bots. It has been suggested that daily administration of pyrantel tartrate may aid in preventing infection with *Sarcosyctis neurona*, the causative organism of equine protozoal myeloencephalitis (EPM).

TARGETED TREATMENT

Only those horses with significant fecal egg counts should be treated to control cyathostomes. The benefit is that this deworming program minimizes use of anthelmintics and encourages the naturally acquired resistance that is developed against the parasites by the immune system.

Management of this program requires regular quantitative fecal egg counts and treatment when cyathostome counts are higher than 100 to 200 eggs per gram of feces (EPG) in order to be effective in minimizing pasture contamination. Stomach bots and tapeworms are not killed by typical dewormers and regular doses normally employed.

This program is not useful in young animals because of the absence of acquired immunity.

STRATEGIC TREATMENT

Strategic treatment deworming is based on the use of effective anthelmintics to eliminate small strongyles in the intestine before the season of the year that is optimal for parasite development in pastures. This approach reduces pasture contamination and thus reinfection of resident horses. It minimizes use of anthelmintics but requires an adequate understanding of the local epidemiology of cyathostome infections. This program may not be as effective in young animals. In northern temperate regions, cyathostome infections have been controlled by treatment administration in the spring, early summer, and fall. In southeastern regions, cyathostome infections may be controlled by beginning these treatments in the early fall. This program can be modified by treating horses with a larvicidal dose of anthelmintic before exposure to pasture during the period of optimal parasite transmission.

CHAPTER 5

Common Internal Parasites of the Horse

LARGE STRONGYLES

These include worms that affect the large intestine, such as *Strongylus vulgaris*, *Strongylus edentatus*, and *Strongylus equinus*. The most damaging parasite of the three is *Strongylus vulgaris* because its immature (larval) forms can migrate through the mesenteric artery in the abdomen and its branches, leading to inflammation of the vessel and development of clots within the artery. Such inflammation can lead to poor blood supply to the intestine and the development of colic, sometimes requiring surgical intervention. Furthermore, heavy burdens of this parasite cause poor growth and anemia. Aberrant migration of these larvae may cause problems in other organ systems.

SMALL STRONGYLES (CYATHOSTOMES)

The major problems caused by cyathostomes are related to the larvae (immature) form of these worms. The larvae can encyst in the mucosal lining of the large intestine, which can lead to chronic colic and poor body condition.

ANOPLOCEPHALA (TAPEWORMS)

Infestations with these worms are usually asymptomatic. However, on rare occasions life-threatening lesions can be associated with these parasites. Various surgical conditions such as cecal-cecal and cecal-colonic intussusception (when the large intestine telescopes into itself or into the colon) have been associated with heavy burdens of these parasites.

ASCARIDS (ROUNDWORMS)

Ascarids can pose problems for foals and yearlings. The major ascarid parasite of horses is *Parascaris equorum*. This parasite has a larval (immature) stage during which the parasites migrate significantly in the portal vein to the liver, then to the heart, lungs, and bronchi and trachea where they are coughed up and swallowed. Foals infested with this parasite can develop coughing, nasal discharge, small intestinal impactions and rupture, and poor growth rates.

STRONGYLOIDES WESTERI (THREADWORMS)

Infection with this parasite is a consideration in foals. The route of infection occurs orally, through the skin, or through transmammary passage of larvae. These worms are, therefore, capable of being transmitted from the dam through her milk to her foal. Prevention of infection in the foal involves appropriate deworming of the mare. Infections are usually self-limiting but could be associated with mild diarrhea in the foal.

GASTEROPHILUS SPECIES (STOMACH BOTS)

These parasites are actually the larval stages of bot flies. The eggs are laid on the coat of the horse, and the larvae migrate to the mouth and are swallowed or migrate to the stomach. They attach to the stomach wall where they may cause ulceration. Perforation of such ulcers occurs rarely.

OXYURIS EQUI (PINWORMS)

These parasites are associated with little significant clinical signs other than tail rubbing and anal irritation. The parasite affects the large intestine, but the female migrates out of the anus to lay eggs, thereby causing the clinical signs of anal irritation.

DICTYOCAULUS ARNFIELDI (LUNGWORM)

This worm is often associated with minimal clinical signs, but it can cause coughing due to parasitic pneumonia in affected horses. Because the parasite is normally found in donkeys, horses that are pastured or stabled with donkeys are at risk of developing respiratory signs associated with this parasite.

STOMACH WORMS

Habronema muscae, Draschia megastoma, and *Trichostrongylus axei* are the major worms affecting the horse's stomach. These worms are often transmitted by flies. They may cause differing clinical syndromes. *Habronema* worms are most commonly associated with "summer sores" on the skin of the horse in response to wound infected with the larvae of this parasite. *Trichostrongylus axei* has been associated with the development of hemorrhagic gastritis. The parasite is carried by cattle; therefore, horses on pasture with cattle may be predisposed to infection. Ivermectin is the treatment of choice for these parasites.

FILARID (*ONCHOCERCA*)

The microfilariae of these species are associated with skin and possibly ocular lesions in the horse. A ventral midline dermatitis in a horse that responds to the administration of ivermectin supports a diagnosis of this condition in association with the *Onchocerca* microfilariae.

EXTERNAL PARASITES

Control of external parasites often requires combined use of pesticides and management to minimize exposure. The control of insect populations where horses are kept requires the use of pesticides and approved formulations on the horse. Directions must be followed carefully to protect horses from toxic effects of these products. Pyrethrins are often used easily and safely in horses.

FLIES

Some biting flies may cause seasonal pruritic dermatitis that appears more severe over mane and tail. Other flies such as *Stomoxys spp.* may cause general irritation and/or disease transmission. Horses may develop hypersensitivity to biting flies manifested as severe itching and hair loss. These species include *Culicoides spp.* and perhaps others. Their control is managed by minimizing exposure to the horses by keeping stalls and pastures relatively clean of manure. Barn screens and/or insecticide spray systems may aid in decreasing exposure within the barn. It helps to turn out with a fly sheet and/or a fly mask during times of the day when flies are least prominent. Spray or wipe-on formulations of pyrethrins are helpful.

LICE

There are two primary species of chewing lice in the horse, *Trichodectes pilosus* and *Damalinia equi*. There is one major species of sucking lice: *Haematopinus asini*. These parasites might cause weight loss, anemia, skin irritation, and general unthriftiness of the affected horse. Lice are best controlled by brushing insecticides into the coat or by high-pressure spray.

MANGE

Dry mange (sarcoptic mange) appears on the belly initially. Wet mange (psoroptic) may begin at the base of the tail and can be fatal. A serous discharge distinguishes this form (wet) from dry mange. Tail or hock mange may be caused by chorioptic mange. Mange can be controlled by intensive application of topical insecticides (weekly) until the skin scrapings from the lesions are negative. Ivermectin is also potentially effective against these parasites. Sarcoptic mange is transmissible to humans and occurs by physical contact.

TICKS

A number of ticks may infect horses. Some species are associated with certain diseases such as the *Ixodes spp.* that are associated with the transmission of Lyme disease to humans and horses alike. Other recognized species of ticks affecting horses include *Otobius megnini, Annocentor nitens*, and *Dermacentor albipictus*, but a number of others are possible. Clinical syndromes possible from tick infestation might include blood loss anemia, depression, and tick paralysis. Chemical pesticides applied as dips and sprays and topical application of ivermectin on the parasite are effective in their individual removal.

MOSQUITOES

Mosquitoes of the *Culex spp.* and others can transmit diseases when they bite susceptible horses. Diseases such as equine infectious anemia; Eastern, Western, and Venezuelan encephalomyelitis; and West Nile virus can be transmitted by mosquitoes. A major requirement in controlling the exposure of horses to mosquitoes appears to be eliminating any standing water in which mosquitoes might reproduce. The use of protective covering, stabling at night, the use of insect repellents, and screened housing will also help reduce exposure to mosquitoes and, thus, their ability to transmit disease to horses.

MANAGEMENT PRACTICES FOR PARASITE CONTROL

Good management practices for an effective parasite control program are essential regardless of the extent and particulars of the deworming program. Good parasite management and control begin with regular evaluation of fecal egg counts. This becomes more important with certain types of deworming programs but is highly advised for all programs. It is ideal for all horses to be dewormed simultaneously and kept on the same schedule. Quarantining of new horses on the farm and preventing fecal contamination of

PERCENT EFFICACY OF VARIOUS DEWORMERS AGAINST COMMON PARASITES

Anthelmintic	Dose (mg/kg)	Safety Index	Class	Anoplocephala	Gasterophilus	P. equorum (roundworms)	Large Strongyles	Small Strongyles	Oxyuris equi (pinworms)	Encysted Small Strongyle larvae	Effective Against Benzimidazole-resistant Small Strongyles
Piperazine	88	17	heterocyclic	ineffective	0	97	5-50	95	50	0	Yes
Thiabendazole	44-88	27	benzimidazole	ineffective	0	42	97	95	95	0	No
Mebendazole	8.8	45	benzimidazole	ineffective	0	97	80-97	87	97	0	No
Fenbendazole	5-10	100	benzimidazole	ineffective	0	95	95-97	97	97	92-96 (10mg/kg; 5days)	No
Oxfendazole	10	10	benzimidazole	ineffective	0	95	97	97	97	0	No
Oxibendazole	10-15	60	benzimidazole	ineffective	0	95	97	97	97	0	No
Levamisole - Piperazine	8 (levamisole) 88 (piperazine)	<3	Imidazothiazole- heterocyclic	ineffective	0	100	63-97	97	90	0	Yes
Pyrantel	6.6	6-20	pyrimidines	effective at 2-3X regular dose**	0	95	70-97	95	65	0	Yes
Trichlorfon	40	1	organophosphate	ineffective	95	97	0	0	95	0	No
Dichlorvos resin pellet	35	3	organophosphate	ineffective	90	97	75-97	90	95	0	Yes
Febantel	6	33	phenylguanidine	ineffective	0	97	97	97	97	0	No
Ivermectin	0.2	10	macrocyclic lactone	ineffective	99	100	100	100	100	35-42	Yes
Moxidectin	0.4	5	macrocyclic lactone	ineffective	90	100	100	100	100	70-80	Yes

water sources also help minimize the exposure of horses to infective stages of parasites.

Pasture management may have tremendous impact on parasite control. Regular cutting of pastures is important to control indirectly the exposure of grazing horses to parasitic larvae. Regular removal of feces from pasture and other areas grazed and populated by horses is helpful to reduce contamination of pastures.

Harrowing pastures to scatter manure and to kill larvae at times of extreme heat and dryness and cold helps reduce pasture contamination. Pasture rotation helps clean pastures at times of the year when larval survival is expected to be minimal. The control of animal density and areas grazed is supported by effective pasture rotation and rest.

CHAPTER 6
Nutrition

GENERAL PRINCIPLES

A complete review of equine nutrition is beyond the scope of this text; however, some basic principles that relate to preventive medicine are worth mentioning. It is always advisable to seek specific suggestions from a nutritionist in developing a feeding program. Feeding programs should meet the individual horse's needs, as these requirements vary with the amount and type of forage and grains fed, amount of pasture available, use of the horse and amount of exercise, and individual metabolism and ambient environmental temperatures. Diets typically should be designed around forage (hay) and grass. Analyzing the hay to identify the amount of energy in calories it provides as well as its mineral content can help achieve a well-designed feeding program. Commercially available grain mixes and pelleted feeds vary to meet the energy and mineral needs of most horses that are used for various types of work or for horses with different needs (performance, broodmares, youth, overweight, geriatric horses).

Another critical component of a feeding program is access to a clean, fresh water source.

Because diets composed entirely of cereal grains are associated with higher risks of diarrhea, colic, acute laminitis, exer-

tional myopathy (tying-up), hyperactivity, and obesity, it is recommended that a grain or concentrate mix make up no more
than half (by weight of dry matter) of the total amount of
feed. Those horses that are less
than one year of age or those
being used for sprint-type exercise may be fed up to 70
percent grain mix, but a
maximum of 50 percent grain
by weight of dry matter of the
diet is generally safer. This
amounts to about one pound
of forage dry matter (weight
corrected for water content)
per 100 pounds of body
weight. Feeding inadequate forage to a horse that is not on
pasture may significantly increase the risk of diarrhea, colic,
founder, wood chewing, feces eating, and in young horses,
mane and tail chewing.

> ## AT A GLANCE
>
> • Feeding programs should meet the individual horse's needs.
>
> • Diets typically should be designed around forage (hay) and grass.
>
> • Grain or concentrate mix should make up no more than half (by weight of dry matter) of the total amount of feed.

Harvested forages should be fed in manners that minimize
forage loss and loss of nutritional value, fecal contamination,
and dust inhalation during consumption. Containers or racks
that catch leaves and loose forage and keep forage off the
ground can be useful. Hay racks, feed troughs, and feed
bunks may serve these purposes. Hay consumption from
feeders or feed bunks that are placed above the horse's
shoulder height increases the likelihood of material getting
into the horse's eyes and dust inhalation while eating. Horses
should be fed individually to assure that each horse gets its
appropriate ration and to reduce competition for these
rations. Hay from round bales is commonly fed but should be
avoided. Feeding round bales is associated with increased incidence of colic, mold spore inhalation that leads to toxin ingestion or the development of chronic respiratory disorders
such as COPD, and increased likelihood of botulism

To help prevent digestive dysfunction, limit grain intake to about 0.5 pounds of grain/100 pounds of body weight per feeding. This grain should be fed to the horse in two to three daily meals. Infrequent meals may induce changes in intestinal motility and blood flow and increase the risk and occurrence of colic, a condition that primarily affects stabled or paddocked horses and is uncommon in horses on pasture. The risk and occurrence of colic in horses that are not on pasture can be reduced by having long-stemmed forage available as much as possible and allowing the horse to eat it freely. Again, long-stemmed hay and pasture should be the basis for all feeding programs. Grain should be fed in as small an amount as possible and only if forage and pasture are unable to meet any additional caloric requirements. The exceptions would include feeding programs for horses with teeth problems that may do better on a complete pelleted feed, or if good-quality forage is unavailable or is considerably more expensive than grain.

Mineral requirements for horses may vary with age, activity, and for the mare, reproductive status. Balance between dietary calcium and phosphorous intake is important for all horses. Growing horses, broodmares in the last trimester of pregnancy, and broodmares that are lactating need more of these minerals. Regardless of the requirement level, these two minerals must be balanced. Diets that fall below an equal ratio of calcium to phosphorous lead to calcium deficiency, which can be caused by inadequate calcium intake or excess phosphorous intake. Clinical disease associated with this condition causes excess parathyroid hormone secretion (known as "nutritional secondary hyperparathyroidism"). Excess parathyroid hormone causes calcium and phosphorous to be mobilized from bone "reserves" and may lead to bone demineralization, enlarged facial bones, shifting leg lameness, and generalized bone and joint pain.

Dietary changes should be gradual, over several days or weeks. Increasing the amount of grain at a rate of no more than 0.5 pounds daily until the desired level is reached is believed to be a safe approach. Faster rates of change may be associated with the development of colic and/or founder. Furthermore, decreases should be gradual for horses on a high-grain diet that are being rested or retired from strenuous training. Horses in regular strenuous exercise that are given a day's rest should receive less grain that day and should have turn-out in an area of sufficient size to allow them to run (unless being rested for an injury). Horses being put on lush green pasture should be given all the hay they are accustomed to receiving before being put out onto the pasture. If possible, the amount of time spent on such pasture should be gradually increased by one hour each day. After the fourth or fifth day, it is usually safe to leave the horse on the pasture. The more plentiful and lush the pasture, the more important these procedures are for safe introduction to the pasture.

FEEDING THE GROWING HORSE

Feeding of young, growing horses requires a higher amount of digestible energy and specific attention to certain nutrients. Young horses frequently need more protein, calcium, phosphorus, zinc, and copper than that available in most grains and forages. Inadequate dietary protein intake in young horses can reduce growth rates. Slower growth rates reduce the need for some of these nutrients, but the mature horse ultimately may be smaller if growth rate is significantly slowed. As normal or faster-than-normal growth rates are reached, a deficiency of one of the aforementioned minerals becomes more likely (calcium, phosphorus, zinc, and copper). If these deficiencies are not prevented, rapid growth and mineral deficiencies may lead to developmental orthopedic diseases such as osteochondritis dissecans (OCD), wobbler's syndrome, or other bone-related problems. Fast growth rates do not lead to increases in mature size.

Horse owners commonly make the mistake of oversupplementing minerals, which can cause problems as well.

1.1) ENERGY REQUIREMENTS IN FEED FOR GROWING HORSES

Digestible Energy in Mcal/lb in Dry Matter Fed	Crude Protein in % of Dry Matter Fed
Nursing foals: 1.5-1.7 in creep feed in addition to milk	16%
Weanling: 1.3	14.5%
Yearling: 1.25	12.5%
2-year-old: 1.15	12%

1.2) DAILY CALORIC REQUIREMENTS OF GROWING HORSES BASED ON EXPECTED MATURE WEIGHT OF 1100 LBS (MCAL/DAY)

Weanling, 4 months	14.4 Mcal/day
Weanling, 6 months	
Moderate Growth	15.0 Mcal/day
Rapid Growth	17.2 Mcal/day
Yearling, 12 months	
Moderate Growth	18.9 Mcal/day
Rapid Growth	21.3 Mcal/day
Yearling, 18 months	
Moderate Growth	19.8 Mcal/day
Rapid Growth	26.6 Mcal/day
2-Year-Old	
Moderate Growth	18.8 Mcal/day
Rapid Growth	26.3 Mcal/day

Unlimited access to trace-mineralized salt high in copper and zinc usually meets the demand for these minerals. In areas of selenium deficiency, selenium in the mineral block may be worthwhile, but over-supplementation of selenium should be carefully avoided. Trace-mineralized salt does not contain calcium and phosphorus. Generally speaking, only if and when the proper amounts of calcium and phosphorus are in the grain mix or in the forage is a growing horse likely to receive the proper amounts of these minerals.

Grain feeding is often necessary to complete the energy demands of the growing horse and to reach the maximum mature size. However, dietary caloric intake must be avoided for the previously outlined reasons. A summary of suggested energy intake and feed content for growing horses is presented in tables 1.1, 1.2, and 1.3. In addition to feeding adequate levels of protein and minerals to make up for the amounts not supplied by the forage alone, use grain mixes high in the amino acid lysine. Inadequate levels of this amino acid may also reduce growth rates. Soybean meal and canola meal are protein sources that are high in lysine and may be added to mixes insufficient in this amino acid.

Weanlings should not be allowed unlimited access to high-quality legume forage such as alfalfa. Unlimited access to such forage results in excess energy intake and increases the likelihood of developmental orthopedic diseases. Weanlings should be restricted to 0.5 pounds of this type of forage per 100 pounds of anticipated mature body weight. Yearlings, in contrast, may be given unlimited access to

1.3) APPROXIMATE DAILY NUTRIENT REQUIREMENTS FOR GROWING HORSES BASED ON EXPECTED MATURE WEIGHT OF 1100 LBS (MCAL/DAY)							
	Protein(g)	Calcium(g)	Phosphorus(g)	Magnesium(g)	Potassium(g)	Vitamin A (in 1000 IU)	Lysine (g)
Weanling, 4 months	720	34	19	3.7	11.3	8	30
Weanling, 6 months							
Moderate growth	750	29	16	4.0	12.7	10	32
Rapid growth	860	36	20	4.3	13.3	10	36
Yearling, 12 months							
Not in training	859	29	16	5.5	17.8	15	36
In training	956	34	19	5.7	18.2	15	40
Yearling, 18 months							
Not in training	893	27	15	6.4	21.1	18	38
In training	1195	36	20	8.6	28.2	18	50
2-Year-Old							
Not in training	800	24	13	7.0	23.1	20	32
In training	1117	34	19	9.8	32.2	20	45

legume and non-legume forages with little risk of the development of orthopedic diseases related to excess dietary energy intake.

FEEDING FOR MAINTENANCE

In addition to access to good-quality water and trace-mineralized salts, idle horses or horses that receive minimal use or exercise will require between 1.5 and 1.75 pounds of average or higher-quality forage per 100 pounds of bodyweight. In such horses grain supplementation is usually unnecessary and may be ill-advised. For optimal performance and health, a horse should receive the amount and quality of feed to maintain moderate body weight without feeding it more than it can or will eat. Mature, average-quality forage may lack adequate protein and/or caloric density, necessitating the supplementation of grain or other forms of protein. Inadequate protein can be corrected or prevented by adding 1.5 to two pounds of a 24 percent to 30 percent protein supplement or by feeding 3.5 to five pounds of a 16 percent protein grain mix, depending on the protein requirements of the horse and the amount of protein in the diet before supplementation. Feeding three to five pounds of alfalfa hay or pellets daily may also correct a protein deficiency.

Whether a horse on an all-forage diet needs supplemental

feed or minerals can be determined by evaluating the nutritional value provided by the forage and available pasture. Horses in regular work are much more likely to require some supplementation of a particular nutrient or mineral, but this also depends on the content of the forage(s) being fed, the pasture contents, and the content in the grain, grain mixes, or pelleted or extruded feeds. Feeding grain to hard-working horses probably helps them meet nutritional needs without creating the need for excessive feed consumption and excessive gastrointestinal fill. Many commercially available pelleted or extruded feeds are termed "complete," in that they are formulated to meet dietary caloric requirements and vitamin and mineral needs in the idle and in the working adult. Specific rations are available for various levels of exercise, for pregnant mares, and for younger horses. A good program designed for horses being used for physical activity might be one that aims at feeding an adequate amount of forage to meet maintenance requirements and providing grain as needed to meet the additional requirements for the physical activity. Some guidelines for feeding are presented in table 1.4. These are, however, only guidelines. Specific feeding programs that account for individual variables relating to feed quality, vitamin and mineral requirements, level of physical activity, and individual variations in metabolism require feed analysis and "fine-tuning" on an individual horse basis.

FEEDING FOR ATHLETIC PERFORMANCE

Performance activities can be thought of in three general categories: endurance or long-distance activity, middle-distance activity, and short-distance or sprint-like activities. Endurance activity lasts for greater than two hours and involves mainly low-intensity, sub-maximal exertion that requires the production of usable energy predominantly from aerobic metabolism. Such activities include endurance ride and competitive trail ride competitions, work horse activity such as that performed by draft or ranch horses, heavily used

1.4) ENERGY REQUIREMENTS IN FEED FOR ADULT HORSES: (MCAL/LB DRY MATTER FED)	
Maintenance	0.9
Light work and breeding stallion	1.5-1.3
Aged horse	1.0
PROTEIN REQUIREMENTS IN FEED FOR ADULT HORSES: (% DRY MATTER FED)	
Maintenance	8
Light work and breeding stallion	10-11
Aged horse	10
DAILY ENERGY REQUIREMENTS OF HORSES (MCAL/1100 LB HORSE)	
Maintenance	16.4 Mcal/1100 lbs/day
Stallions (breeding)	20.5 Mcal/1100 lbs/day

1.5) APPROXIMATE DAILY NUTRIENT REQUIREMENTS FOR WORKING HORSES (IN GRAMS)						
	Protein (g)	Calcium(g)	Phosphorus(g)	Magnesium(g)	Potassium (g)	Vitamin A (in 1000 IU)
Light work	820	25	18	9.4	31.2	22
Moderate work	984	30	21	11.3	37.4	22
Intense work	1312	40	29	15.1	49.9	22

1.6) APPROXIMATE CALORIC REQUIREMENTS FOR WORKING HORSES	
Light work	20.5 Mcal/1100 lbs/day
Moderate work	24.6 Mcal/1100 lbs/day
Intense work	32.8 Mcal/1100 lbs/day
APPROXIMATE GRAIN REQUIRED FOR PHYSICAL ACTIVITY	
Light activity (pleasure riding)	0.5-1.5 lbs grain per hour of activity
Moderate activity	2-3 lbs grain per hour of activity
Strenuous activity	4 or more lbs per hour of activity

school horses for riding lessons, and upper-level, heavily campaigned show horse and three-day event activity. Middle-distance performance involves the exertion of the horse at an average of 75 percent to 95 percent of maximal intensity for several minutes. Distance equivalents may range from one-half to two miles, depending on the intensity of exertion. This type of exercise frequently uses both aerobic and anaerobic metabolism. It would include most racing performed by Standardbred and Thoroughbred horses. Finally, maximal exertion for a minute or less is associated with primarily anaerobic metabolism. It would be expected in horses sprinting a distance of a half-mile or less. Such activity is seen with Quarter Horse racing, barrel racing, rodeo events, and draft horse pulling competitions.

To meet the daily energy requirements for horses in any of the above levels of physical activity, grain should be offered only in amounts that compensate for the extent to which caloric intake supplied by forage is exceeded by energy requirements for the physical activity. This is best estimated by having a feed analysis performed and estimating the amount of forage eaten by the animal and knowing the forage's caloric density. Mineral and vitamin requirements must be met as well. Such requirements may be met most accurately and cost-effectively by knowing what the requirements are for the horse at its level of performance and by evaluating the forage content and grain, grain mix, or pellets fed for these nutrients. Furthermore, it must be known how much of each feed type the horse consumes. Many horses may not require further supplementation of most nutrients if they are eating high-quality green forage. Even protein requirements may be met in a majority of horses by providing the appropriate grain ration and by having adequate amounts of high-quality forage in the diet; for example, alfalfa hay is quite high in protein (perhaps 17 percent to 20 percent), calcium, and phosphorus. Alfalfa may, however, be associated with loose manure and laminitis if it is not fed in an appropriate amounts adjusted to the individual horse. The amount of minerals, vitamins, and crude protein in hay is greatest if the hay is harvested and cured before reaching maturity. After maturity (flowering or coming to seed) the forages that are harvested for hay are significantly reduced in protein, vitamin, and mineral content. Grazing on growing grasses may also provide substantial amounts of calories, protein, calcium, and phosphorus, further reducing the requirements from other feedstuffs. The amount grass contributes to the diet for various nutrients can be estimated from tables of the approximate contents for each grass type or, more accurately, by submitting a sample of the grass forage for specific analysis. Tables 1.5 and 1.6 are provided as guidelines only. Specific needs of any horse should be evaluated individually relative to the level and intensity of activities performed and individual variability.

FEEDING DURING PREGNANCY AND LACTATION

Throughout usually the first seven to eight months of gestation, the nutritional requirements of the pregnant mare do not differ substantially from that of idle horses. In fact, the nutritional requirements of barren and non-lactating mares may be

1.7) APPROXIMATE CALORIC REQUIREMENTS FOR PREGNANT AND LACTATING MARES BASED ON 1100 LBS MATURE WEIGHT OF MARE

Pregnant mares	
9 months	18.2 Mcal/1100 lbs/day
10 months	18.5 Mcal/1100 lbs/day
11 months	19.7 Mcal/1100 lbs/day
Lactating mares	
Foaling to 3 months	28.3 Mcal/1100 lbs/day
3 months to weaning	24.3 Mcal/1100 lbs/day

1.8) NUTRIENT REQUIREMENT IN FEED (% DRY MATTER)

	Protein %	Calcium %	Phosphorus %
Nonlactation and prior to the last 3 months of pregnancy	8	0.25	0.20
Last 3 months of pregnancy	11	0.50	0.35
Lactation	13	0.50	0.35

1.9) ENERGY REQUIREMENTS IN FEED FOR BROODMARES (MCAL/LB DRY MATTER FED)

Nonlactation and before last 3 months of pregnancy	0.9 Mcal/lb feed
Last 3 months of pregnancy	1.0-1.1 Mcal/lb feed
Lactation	1.1 Mcal/lb feed

met by feeding forage with greater than eight percent protein by dry weight and providing access to trace-mineralized salt up to the final trimester of pregnancy (last three to four months). During the last trimester and during lactation, the requirements for dietary energy, protein, calcium, and phosphorus increase significantly. During the final trimester and during lactation, nutrient requirements may be met by feeding a forage greater than 11 percent by dry weight in protein and providing access to trace-mineralized salt fortified with calcium and phosphorous. If a forage less than 11 percent protein is fed, the diet may be supplemented with a grain or pelleted mix as needed.

Dietary energy requirements increase progressively, 10 percent to 20 percent during gestation and 80 percent during lactation. Inadequate energy consumption may cause a decrease in milk production and reproductive efficiency. For mares to maintain body weight during pregnancy, their weight must increase by an amount equal to the foal's birth weight plus the weight of the placenta and fluids (about nine percent to 12 percent of the mare's weight). For the 1,100-pound mare, the total gain should be between 100 and 130 pounds during pregnancy with 0.75 to 1 pound gained daily during the last 90 days of pregnancy. Tables 1.7, 1.8, and 1.9 are meant as guidelines for the requirements during pregnancy and lactation. A complete feed analysis and evaluation of individual nutrient needs are best performed on an individual basis.

THE UNDERWEIGHT HORSE

Managing and caring for a persistently underweight horse can be difficult and frustrating for the owner and/or caretaker. A number of factors can be involved or contribute to the condition. A primary and initial evaluation should focus on the basics of nutrition. Ascertaining the animal's appetite, the quality of feed provided, and the available quantity can help determine whether there is nutritional inadequacy that can be corrected. Caloric supplementation may be all that is required to regain and maintain adequate body condition. Addition of corn oil, a fat supplement, or another calorically dense feed may meet this need. For older horses, after an oral examination has ruled out significant dental problems, switching to a more easily digestible feed formulated for older horses may be warranted.

Another factor that might lead to inadequate caloric or nutrient intake could be activity or stress that exceeds the horse's diet. A feed analysis and a reduction in stress and/or activity might be necessary. The next consideration is that of gastrointestinal parasitism, including the possibility of the presence of larval stages of the parasites and/or encysted stages of small strongyles (cyathostomes) that are prohibiting the animal from thriving. A good oral examination should also be performed to rule out problems related to the horse's mouth and/or dentition. This becomes a significant consideration in aged horses that have worn and erupted the full extent of their dentition and no longer have teeth capable of occlusion or mastication of feeds. Such instances might require "slurry diets" to ensure adequate nutrition. Furthermore, such horses with poor dentition may be at greater risk for esophageal choke and colic due to poor mastication. Horses in regular performance or in stressful situations such as overcrowding may suffer from gastrointestinal ulceration. Medical therapy of such conditions using specific anti-ulcer medications is effective in resolving clinical signs and pathology caused by gastrointestinal ulcers. Feed digestibility can become a significant factor in older horses. Therefore, feed changes to a more digestible diet such as commercially produced geriatric feeds may be necessary.

Once feed analysis has been fully evaluated, other causes of poor condition must be considered. Chronic disease conditions, chronic causes of colic or malabsorption, and gastric and duodenal and/or colonic ulceration should be considered. Evaluating horses for such conditions may become difficult and costly. Such evaluation will require veterinary intervention and evaluation.

CHAPTER 7
Using Dietary Supplements

The use of dietary supplements in horses has exploded over the past several years, creating a big and profitable market for these types of products. As this market has exploded, so has the advertisement and promotion of these products. Indeed, it is becoming more and more difficult to find horses that are not receiving a "supplement" of some type. Although numerous supplements are specifically and appropriately designed to meet certain needs or for certain conditions, the impression of how often these supplements are needed may be inflated in some, if not many, instances. Using unnecessary supplements becomes very expensive over time. Indeed, the provision of excess dietary supplements may be harmful to the health and performance of a horse. The vitamin, mineral, protein, and other nutritional needs of each horse should be evaluated based on the function of the animal or its level of work. The major reasons that I encounter indiscriminate dietary supplementation include the following:

- overestimation of the horse's level of work
- overestimation of the dietary and nutrient requirements for the level of work being performed
- a feeling supplementation is needed because everyone else seems to be giving some supplement without adequate evaluation of the dietary needs versus activity level.

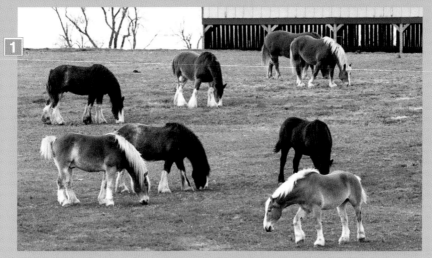

Housing horses by age and function can minimize the spread of disease (1).

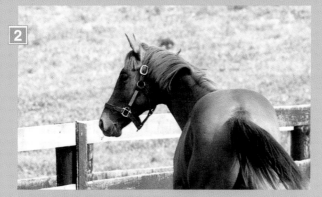

It is sometimes necessary to isolate a horse (2).
Negative Coggins tests should accompany all newly
arriving horses (3).

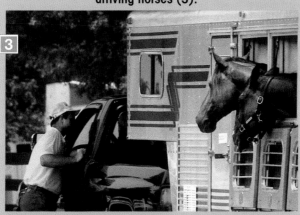

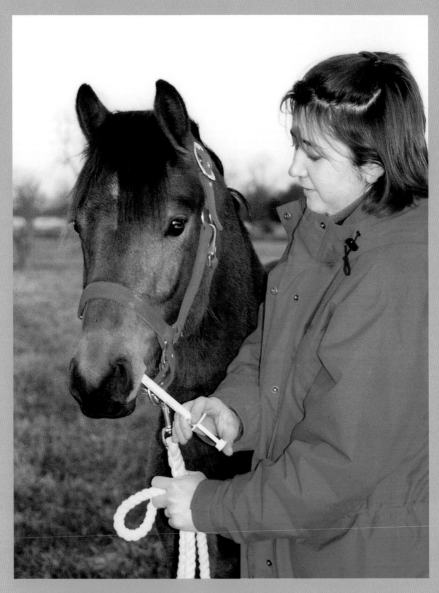

Foals can be susceptible to several parasites. Consult with a veterinarian about a deworming program. Opposite: some vaccines are administered intramuscularly; others, via the nostril.

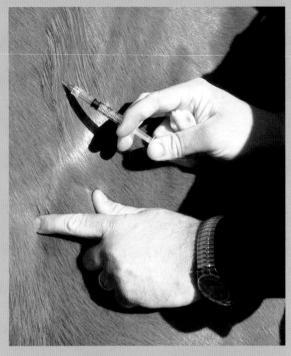

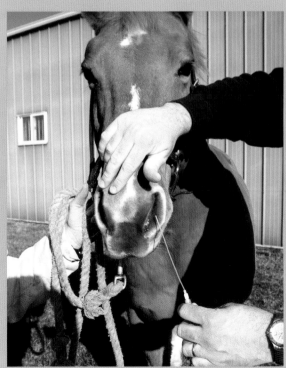

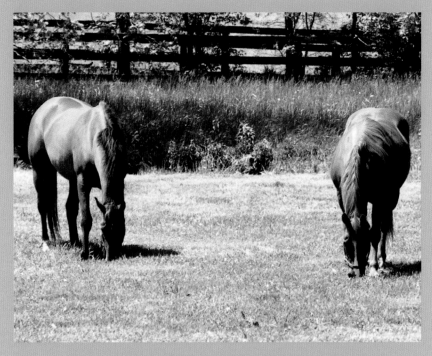

Forages — grass and hay — should compose all or most of a horse's diet.

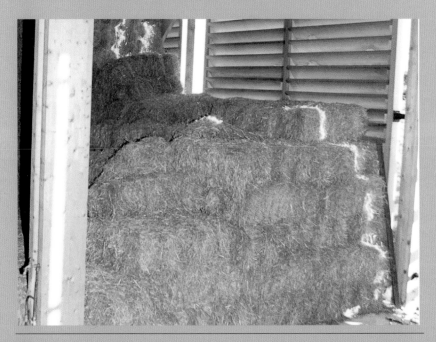

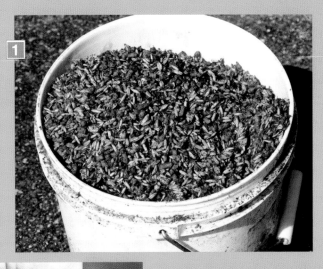

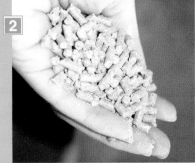

Commercially available grain mixes
and pelleted feeds (1 & 2) can
augment some horses' diets.
Moistening feed can make it easier to
chew for older horses.

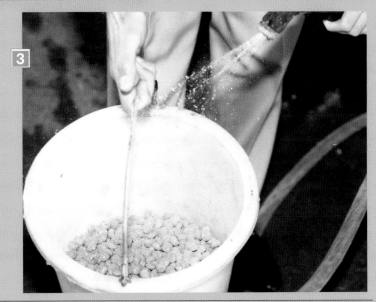

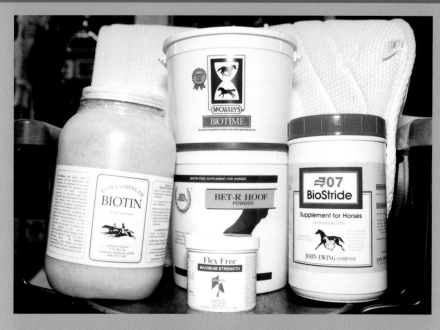

There are numerous supplements for feet on the market (above).

The use of joint supplements in performance horses is increasing.

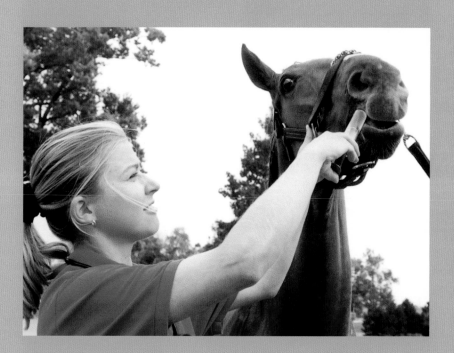

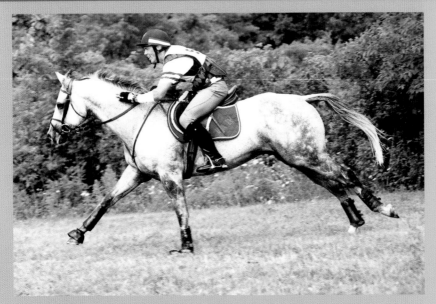

No horse can be expected to perform at the same level over the years. Arthritic changes are normal, and many horses can still be useful at a lower level of activity.

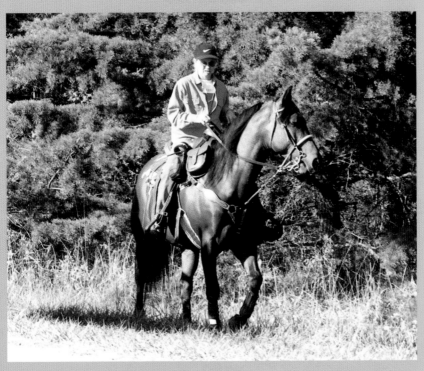

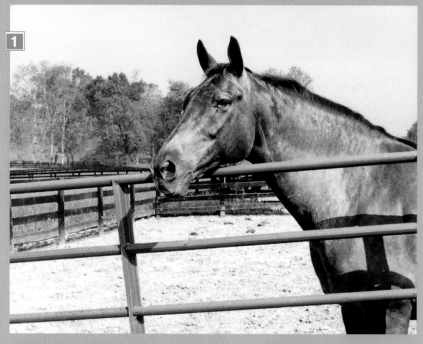

Overweight horses need to be put on strict diets to avoid episodes or recurrence of laminitis (1). The veterinarian flexes the front and hind legs (2 & 3) as part of a physical examination.

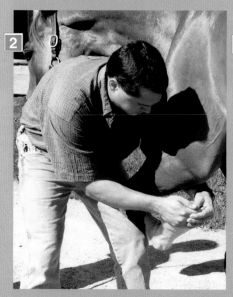

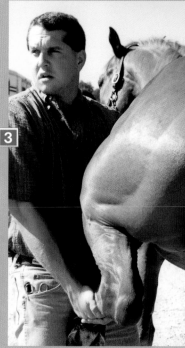

- a feeling that it is a means of providing the horse the very best of care and nutrition.

Many, if not most, horses' dietary requirements can be met with a well-formulated diet that includes good pasture and/or high-quality hay and well-formulated commercial feeds that are used appropriately to account for the shortcomings (if any) of the forage component. For these reasons, have a good grasp of your individual horse's needs based on its activity level and what its diet

> ## AT A GLANCE
>
> - Many horses' dietary requirements can be met with a well-formulated feed plan.
>
> - Careful consideration of a horse's needs should be given before adding supplements to its diet.
>
> - Benefits from joint supplements may only be realized with regular use over an extended period.

provides before you add a nutritional supplement. Secondly, go through the above four points and honestly decide if any of them influence your desire to add a supplement. Nutritional supplements are most likely to be useful and indicated when a feed and pasture analysis indicates a deficiency of a particular nutrient in the diet, when the horse is growing, when broodmares are in the last three months of gestation or lactating, or when the horse is performing athletically with significant intensity.

PROTEIN, VITAMINS, AND MINERALS

Daily dietary protein, vitamin, and mineral requirements are best met for most horses by high-quality grass or legume hay (alfalfa) and good pasture. When a horse is without access to good pasture, these requirements can be provided by forage hay and/or the grain or pelleted ration. Horses without access to good pasture and/or to good hay are much more likely to require specific supplementation of a number of these nutrients. Horses used heavily or used for unusually intense or strenuous activity might also require supplementation even when receiving good pasture and hay. In the chapter on nutrition, you can get an idea of your horse's requirements based on its activity level. Remember that the need for supplementation must be evaluated by knowing what amount of the requirement is met by the feeding program. Do not oversupplement; oversupplementation is wasteful, expensive, and potentially harmful.

FAT SUPPLEMENTATION

Horses engaged in severe exercise or competition, lactating or pregnant mares, and growing horses may require additional calories from grain or pelleted feed because those food sources' energy density is greater than that of forages. High-fat diets benefit horses used for athletic performance by 1) increasing the energy density of a diet without requiring a proportionate increase in the amount of feed required, 2) decreasing the amount of energy used for heat production, 3) increasing the amount of muscle glycogen content, if high-fat diets (up to 10 percent to 12 percent fat added to the total diet) are fed for a sufficient amount of time; 4) improving use of muscle glycogen during anaerobic activity and conserving muscle glycogen during aerobic activity. High-fat diets appear beneficial for both sprint and endurance exercise.

Including up to 20 percent added fat to the total diet and 30 percent in the grain mix may increase caloric density. Horses cannot use more fat content than this without increasing the risk of adverse effects. Fat supplementation may be required with lactating or pregnant mares, horses in extremely demanding competition or exercise, or horses that are not gaining or maintaining weight well. One pint of a fat oil such as corn oil or canola oil may be added per five pounds of grain and results in 20 percent fat added to the total diet. If half the total diet by weight is grain, adding this same amount of fat to the grain will result in adding 10 percent fat to the diet. If one half of the diet is not grain, the amount of fat added should be adjusted so that the total diet does not contain more than 10 percent to 12 percent added fat.

SUPPLEMENTS FOR MUSCLE

A number of supplements are promoted as increasing strength and muscle endurance during exercise. Some of these supplements are directed at buffering or helping to remove the build-up of lactic acid that occurs with anaerobic conditions in muscle. Such conditions exist in muscle tissue when the supply of oxygen can't keep up with the intensity or duration of exercise. Other supplements are designed to "improve blood flow" to working muscle or to provide extra sources of energy storage in the form of muscle creatine (phosphocreatine) under the assumption that such energy will improve the strength and decrease the "fatigue" or time to fatigue for muscle. Despite individual testimonials for these products, their use may be based on faulty understanding of muscle physiology. Under scientific evaluation, these products often fall short of having defendable clinical efficacy. Individual testimonials often do not account for the potential benefits of training, feeding, and other therapies that horses may be concurrently receiving. Nevertheless, some owners and trainers have confidence in some products of this nature. If cost is a concern, it may be more prudent to invest in other areas or products with significant scientific backing.

Vitamin E and selenium are often used as supplements both by oral administration and by injection. However, many horses that receive supplementation, particularly of selenium, may not benefit from it, as they are not living in selenium-deficient areas. Vitamin E appears to be a reasonable supplement for performance horses. However, evaluation of selenium levels in the diet would be warranted before supplementation since oversupplementation causes poor hoof, mane, and tail growth and condition.

SUPPLEMENTS FOR THE THYROID GLAND

Thyroid disease is commonly treated in equine practice despite significant shortcomings in diagnosis. Most practitioners use serum T3 and T4 values as indicators of thyroid disease. Not uncommonly, trainers request such testing under the auspices of being able to diagnose hypothyroidism accurately, using these levels to indicate thyroid disease. Unfortunately, such testing is not very helpful in the specific diagnosis of hypothyroidism in the horse, and the interpretation of these T3 and T4 values is much more complicated than simply determining whether the measured values fall below the "range of normal" provided by the laboratory. Things that affect thyroid level values for T3 and T4 include normal diurnal variation of these levels, sampling time relative to meal intake, illness and/or stress, and medications that the horse is receiving (such as phenylbutazone). These variables significantly alter T3 and T4 levels and make single and even repeat serum T3 and T4 levels relatively unhelpful in diagnosing thyroid disease and hypothyroidism. Specific diagnosis of hypothyroidism requires the administration of thyroid stimulating hormone (TSH) or thyroid releasing hormone (TRH) and sampling of the subsequent thyroid hormone levels in response to such stimulation. Despite the impression one may receive from the number of horses and ponies receiving thyroid supplementation, true adult hypothyroidism occurs infrequently and is generally not life-threatening in itself. Hypothyroidism in the foal is cause for more concern. In foals, it is believed to be related to nutritionally inadequate or excessive intake of iodine by the dam. Goiter (enlargement of the thyroid gland) may be seen with inadequate intake of iodine in adults and may be seen in foals born to mares receiving excessive amounts of iodine in their diet. For adult horses, the National Research Council recommends a daily iodine intake of 0.1 mg/kg of feed, or a total daily intake of 1 to 2 milligrams of iodine per horse.

SUPPLEMENTS FOR JOINTS

In the past several years there has been an explosion of supplements marketed as protecting and maintaining joint health. Early in the development of these products, information regarding their labeled usage was limited. However, increasing amounts of scientific information suggest that regular use of such products may be beneficial.

By far, the most common compounds included in joint supplements include chondroitin sulfate and glucosamine. There is skepticism that these products can be given orally and somehow be broken down in the horse's digestive tract into something that can be used to improve the health of joints. There is a theory why chondroitin sulfate can be used by the horse to improve the joint environment. When chondroitin sulfate breaks down in the horse's body, it probably produces a compound or by-product that can be absorbed by the horse. This compound has a low molecular weight (which can be better absorbed by the horse). These low molecular weight products may, however, have biologic activity, and numerous positive clinical responses to oral supplementation with chondroitin sulfate have been reported.

Glusosamine is another commonly used compound in oral joint supplements. This compound exists as a small, water-soluble molecule that the intestine can easily absorb. Researchers who have examined this compound have found an affinity for joint cartilage and that this compound genuinely appears to modify disease processes in the joint. There appears to be anti-inflammatory activity and the suggestion of the ability to help reverse cartilage degradation in human patients. The information suggests that glucosamine is the most logical choice for the treatment and prevention of joint disease in horses. It is estimated that a 10g/day oral dosage is necessary for a 500kg (1,100 pounds) horse.

Joint supplements that contain the compounds described above may help maintain and sustain joint health. Glucosamine may also help repair cartilage damage to an extent. However, one should not be under the impression that providing such supplements will effectively cure joint disease in the horse. The benefits from joint supplements may only be realized with regular use and over an extended period. Any degenerative joint disease that may exist in a horse should be considered a condition that cannot be specifically cured. The use of oral joint supplements may help to slow the degradation and deterioration of the joint with extended use of these products, but the disease will continue to progress. Successful management of such disease might be prolonged by the use of oral joint supplements with or without other joint therapies.

SUPPLEMENTS FOR THE SKIN AND COAT

It has been suggested for a number of years that feeding high amounts of unsaturated fats increases the oil produced by the skin, giving the horse a shinier coat. However, supporting evidence is lacking. Nonetheless, many owners, trainers, and veterinarians advocate the addition of corn, safflower, or soy oil to the feed to provide a glossy coat. Many individual testimonials support such practice. Because such supplementation is generally safe and inexpensive, it may be worthwhile to consider when other causes of poor coat such as dermatological problems or systemic illnesses are carefully ruled out.

HOOF SUPPLEMENTS

A number of nutritional factors are promoted as hoof growth aids. Such products may include gelatin, numerous vitamins, minerals, amino acids, and other dietary supplements. However, if a horse's nutritional requirements are being met with good-quality forage, grain, or pellets, none of these supplements have shown significant effect on hoof growth.

However, feeding extra biotin may benefit horses with thin, brittle hoof walls, crumbling hoof walls, and/or thin, tender soles. Biotin is therefore recommended for such hoof defects at a dose of 1.2 to 1.5 mg/100 lbs of body weight daily. Smaller doses of 0.10 to 0.15 mg/100 lbs of body weight or 0.1 mg/ lb of total diet may help maintain good hoof structure and prevent the recurrence of hoof problems in horses. Generally speaking, one should also try to ensure that the diet fed meets the protein and calcium requirements of the individual horse based on its athletic use or other function. Oversupplementation with protein and/or calcium may be associated with other health problems.

SUPPLEMENTS OF BENEFIT TO THE PERFORMANCE HORSE (WHEN USED APPROPRIATELY)

An increase in exercise also directly increases the needs for vitamins A, E, B-1, and for folic acid. Vitamin E and selenium supplementation may help decrease oxidative damage from energy production. Adding 1mg of selenium and 1,000 IU of vitamin E to the daily diet may provide selenium and vitamin E supplementation. Only using salt mixes that contain selenium is an alternative way of providing the element. A balanced vitamin supplement may best provide the additional needed vitamins. However, once again, it is important not to overestimate the intensity of exercise and competition your horse performs so that you do not oversupplement with potentially harmful levels of these additives and you do not waste money.

Support of the need for or benefit of a number of commonly used supplements appears limited. Hematinics or "blood builders" such as iron or vitamin B-12 and vitamin C do not appear to provide any benefit to performance horses. Administration of such vitamins and minerals may be best reserved for specific instances when a deficiency of these dietary elements is diagnosed. Several other supplements routinely used to benefit performance horses have little or no evidence supporting their use. Some of these include MSM (methyl sulfonyl methane), DMSO (dimethylsulfoxide), octacosanol, the enzyme super oxide dismutase (SOD), gamma hydroxybutyrate, gamma oryzanol, bioflavonoids, inosine and carnitine, pangamic acid, and some drugs such as nandrolone and amphetamine. Despite lacking scientific support, some have received significant testimonial backing. Of these compounds, MSM and DMSO apparently received significant support from many laypeople and many veterinarians.

CHAPTER 8

Musculoskeletal Maintenance

M aintaining musculoskeletal health is important for horses engaged in competition or exercise activity of any sort. As a horse ages, the incidence of musculoskeletal disorders such as osteoarthritis is likely to increase. Therefore, it may become necessary to manage these problems in order to maintain the best possible performance from such horses. Musculoskeletal problems are not limited to joint disease or arthritis. Indeed, a number of possible problems can be associated with the muscle itself. The incidence of muscular problems may be less common than that of skeletal problems, but muscle problems may require specific and intensive management to assure peak performance.

The overall management and maintenance of musculoskeletal problems and well being include a number of treatments ranging from rest, pharmacotherapy (the use of medications), physical therapy, and other complementary therapies.

MUSCLE MAINTENANCE/TYING-UP SYNDROMES

Probably the most commonly encountered muscle problem in performance horses involves the acute or chronic condition known as "tying-up." During such episodes, muscles become stiff and painful to the horse as a result of muscle damage. The specific cause or causes of this syndrome are often unclear. Suggested causes have included vitamin E/selenium deficiency, hormonal imbalances, hypothyroidism, electrolyte depletion or imbalance, accumulation of lactic acid, extremes of weather, metabolic abnormalities such as specific glycogen storage diseases, and certain viral infections. Some of these speculated causes have received more scientific support than others. For example, no significant evidence links hypothyroidism to tying-up, and indeed true hypothyroidism appears to be fairly uncommon in horses (see Chapter 7). A common

AT A GLANCE

- Tying-up is the most commonly encountered muscle problem in performance horses.

- The gradual progression of degenerative joint disease is normal and expected and can be managed in most cases.

- NSAIDs are extremely useful medications for performance and exercising horses.

cause of tying-up is overuse of an unfit horse. Therefore, adequate training and preparation for exercise and competition will also be valuable in preventing this syndrome.

Recently, there has been extensive investigation into congenital and heritable glycogen storage diseases that are found particularly in the Quarter Horse breed. Such diseases usually cause moderate to severe episodes of tying-up in young and old horses affected with the disease(s). A muscle biopsy is often required to diagnose the disease. Horses with these conditions should be kept from breeding. Management of horses that are affected with such diseases usually requires high-fat diets. Restriction of exercise becomes necessary in horses that are significantly affected. A particular form of glycogen storage disease is called glycogen branching enzyme deficiency. To date, this disease appears to affect very young foals and generally to be fatal or lead to euthanasia.

The diagnosis of tying-up syndrome primarily relies on the recognition of clinical signs of muscle pain and stiffness and identifying increases in serum activity of muscle enzymes such as CK, AST, and LDH. However, correct interpretation of elevation of these enzymes can be less than straightforward.

Such muscle enzymes may increase mildly after exercise. Other horses that are severely cramped or "tied-up" may exhibit lower enzyme activities than horses with milder signs. A diagnosis should not be based on the criteria of muscle enzymes that fall out of the "normal range" provided by the laboratory. True evidence of tying-up is often associated with both clinical signs and with elevations of all the muscle enzymes into the tens and hundreds of thousands. Supplements for the "prevention" of this syndrome are generally unrewarding. Some preventive treatments that have been advocated include the administration of Dantrolene®, electrolytes and sodium bicarbonate, vitamin E/ selenium, Lactanase®, dimethylglycine (DMG), Rubeola Virus Immunomodulator (RVI®), altrenogest in fillies (Regumate®), low-dose tranquilization, and phenytoin. No published studies support the clinical efficacy of most of these treatments in preventing or treating tying-up. Vitamin E and selenium supplementation are likely to help when these nutrients are lacking in the diet. However, phenytoin has received some scientific support for the prevention of tying-up. Concurrent administration of other drugs with phenytoin can produce undesirable side effects. Therapeutic levels should be monitored to prevent such side effects. This medication may best be used if and when other therapies have failed. Treatment with phenytoin should be considered and administered only with the guidance of a veterinarian.

JOINT MAINTENANCE

Equine athletes are really no different than human athletes in regard to the effects of aging, exercise, and other use on the joints. Because this is the case, if a horse is used for regular performance, competition, or other exercise activity, one should see changes over a period of time relating to the joints and skeletal system. Indeed, even aging itself can lead to deterioration in such structures. It is therefore important that an owner and trainer understand that no individual horse can or should be expected to compete at the same level throughout its entire life and that gradual progression of degenerative joint disease and musculoskeletal deterioration are normal and expected. However, today we are armed with a number of potentially useful and some highly proven therapies that can be used to prolong both the length of time a horse is able to compete at its highest potential level and the amount of time that a horse is able to perform the particular activity with comfort and success.

There are a number of modes of therapy that can help maintain joint health and reduce pain associated with joint disease. Such therapies may include oral medications, oral joint supplements, intramuscular medications, intravenous medications, and intra-articular medications (medications that are placed directly into the joint). Other therapies include magnetic therapy, acupuncture, topically administered medications, shock-wave therapy, and more.

JOINT SUPPLEMENTS

This topic was covered in Chapter 7 of this book. A brief address here is appropriate. Oral joint supplements are primarily composed of two compounds: chondroitin sulfate and glucosamine. Adding the supplement to the feed once or twice a day often provides regular administration of these compounds. Oral joint supplements have received numerous positive testimonials for their use. However, one should be reminded that degenerative joint disease cannot be cured and these oral products probably do not impact joint health unless they are used regularly for extended periods.

The use of these compounds, particularly glucosamine, to maintain joint health has some scientific support. A reasonable approach to these oral products may best be reached if one considers such therapy potentially helpful in maintaining joint health and in possibly slowing degenerative joint disease, thereby prolonging the performance life of the animal and its comfort.

SYSTEMIC ANTI-INFLAMMATORY AGENTS

A number of commonly used systemic anti-inflammatory medications are on the market. In a very broad sense, two categories may be identified. The first category may be termed the non-steroidal anti-inflammatory drugs (NSAIDs), and the second is the steroidal anti-inflammatory drugs. These drugs are primarily used to treat pain and inflammation associated with acute injuries or for acute pain and inflammation associated with a chronic injury or condition. In some instances such medications may also be used before a competition or other exercise to prevent pain associated with chronic conditions. The operative word in the description of the use of these medications is "acute." These medications cannot be safely administered for extended periods of time without significantly increasing the risk of their side effects. Therefore, they are usually used to control acute pain for a finite period, until other therapies can specifically address the *cause of the pain*. Again, an exception to this occurs when these medications are used before a specific event or period of exercise. In such instances, the medications are administered on a one-time basis in accordance with the rules specified by USA Equestrian, the racing commission, or some other regulating body.

NSAIDs are extremely useful medications for performance and exercising horses. They are probably much more commonly used than steroidal anti-inflammatory drugs. NSAIDs commonly administered for the control of pain and inflammation include the following: Banamine® (flunixin meglumine), bute (Phenylbutazone), Ketofen® (ketoprofen), naproxen, Arquel® (meclofenamic acid), and others. These medications are important and powerful agents used to combat pain and inflammation. However, they must be used judiciously to minimize potential side effects associated with prolonged usage. Prolonged use of these medications can lead to kidney and gastrointestinal disorders. They are safe to use when appropriately administered under a veterinarian's recommendation.

Steroids are used slightly less for musculoskeletal disease.

These medications tend to be extremely potent anti-inflammatory agents. Steroidal anti-inflammatory medications must be used very carefully as prolonged usage and high doses can suppress normal immune system functions and the horse's production of natural circulating steroids, which are necessary for normal body mechanisms. Furthermore, a number of sources suggest an association between certain steroids and laminitis in horses. Although cause and effect in the development of laminitis is not scientifically substantiated, there does appear to be a cause for concern. For this and the other reasons already mentioned, caution in using these medications is well warranted.

Steroidal therapy is generally regarded as undesirable when the cause of the pain and inflammation is associated with infection. However, in some instances steroids are used *in combination* with antibiotics to help resolve severe inflammation associated with an infection. Examples of steroid anti-inflammatory drugs include dexamethasone (Azium®), betamethasone (Celestone®), flumethasone (Flucort®), prednisolone (Depo-medrol®), triamcinolone (Vetalog®), and others.

INTRAVENOUSLY (IV) AND INTRAMUSCULARLY (IM) ADMINISTERED JOINT THERAPIES

As is the case with oral joint supplements, the availability and use of IV- and IM-administered joint medications have expanded significantly in the past several years. Such therapies often include hyaluronic acid (HA) preparations (e.g., Legend® and others) and polysulfated glycosaminoglycans (PSGAGs) (e.g., Adequan® IM). Hyaluronic acid preparations can be administered intravenously as well as directly into the joint. In the joint, HA performs several functions, such as increasing the viscosity of joint fluid, lubricating the joint membrane and joint cartilage, and other potentially significant functions. Administering HA to a joint is believed to increase the viscosity of normal joint fluid and counter inflammation.

The effects of HA in a joint are maximized by direct injection; however, there is some evidence that intravenous administration of HA may effectively manage osteoarthritis (degenerative joint disease).

PSGAG preparations are most often administered into the muscle, but preparations for direct joint injection are also frequently used. PSGAGs incorporate into the complex molecule that constitutes part of the joint cartilage matrix, decrease the activity of enzymes that cause degradation of joint cartilage, and increase the production of HA and other beneficial molecules in the joint.

Though these therapies tend to be more expensive than oral joint supplements, evidence shows they, too, support and maintain healthy joint cartilage. How expensive the medications are depends on how often they are used. As in the case of oral supplementation for joints, the utility of injectable joint therapies might be improved with regular and prolonged use. These medications do not cure degenerative joint disease but may aid in slowing disease progression and in maintaining normal joint cartilage. They are best used to help prevent and manage osteoarthritis (degenerative joint disease).

INTRA-ARTICULAR THERAPIES (MEDICATIONS ADMINISTERED INTO THE JOINT)

With years of performance, or when there are underlying and perhaps chronic joint problems, medications administered orally or by IM and/or IV injection may become inadequate to provide prolonged relief of joint pain. This leads to reduction in performance for that animal. When this occurs, a specific lameness examination is advisable to identify the affected joint(s). This is typically done by your veterinarian with the use of flexion tests, nerve blocks, joint blocks, radiography, ultrasound examination, and/or other diagnostic imaging techniques. If joint disease is diagnosed, intra-articular therapies (joint injections) should be considered.

A number of people strongly object to joint injections.

Their staunch opposition may have stemmed from the barrage of research specifically on the use of steroids in joints that emerged in the late 1960s and '70s. This research emphasized the potential for adverse effects of corticosteroids on joint cartilage. The incidence of these adverse effects is probably increased by frequent and repetitive use of steroids in a joint with significant underlying problems and continued athletic exercise. A steroid's potency and individual characteristics may impact the likelihood of negative effects on cartilage when used frequently and when athletic use is continued at the same level.

Despite the obvious stigma left from this information regarding steroidal joint injections, appropriate veterinary administration of this therapy can greatly reduce potential for negative effects.

Furthermore, not all joint therapies use steroids. In fact, hyaluronic acid (HA) and polysulfated glycosaminoglycans (PSGAGs) have also been regularly and safely administered into joints. Administration of HA and PSGAGs into a joint helps control inflammation. Your veterinarian will diagnose any joint problem that may exist and determine the best way to manage the condition. For instance, a bone chip in an ankle might require surgery followed by regular maintenance therapy with intramuscular administration of PSGAGs for several weeks after surgery and at regular intervals thereafter. For degenerative joint disease, your veterinarian may be able to control pain and inflammation with intermittent anti-inflammatory medications and/or other joint therapy for a prolonged time. Progression of the disease might require more intensive therapy with hyaluronic acid and/or PSGAGs. Depending on the progression and the costs of non-articular therapies, joint injections may be the most practical and effective way to control the problem.

The type of steroid should be selected with care and is best left to your veterinarian. Frequently, steroids are mixed with hyaluronic acid or steroid types are mixed with one another.

For instance, a "short-acting" steroid may be mixed with a "long-acting" steroid. Commonly affected joints that can be relatively easily injected include the coffin joints, fetlock joints, carpal joints (knee), pastern joint, stifle joints, and hock joints. A single administration of a steroid into a joint is commonly effective for many months and occasionally much longer. It may be most practical and most effective to consider this therapy over others. The longevity of the clinical effect will be important to monitor along with re-evaluation of "soundness" and X-rays to follow the disease's progression. It is probably more fair and humane to the performance horse to administer intra-articular steroids than to force the animal to perform in pain continually with poor results. Many horses can continue for years using judiciously administered steroidal joint injections. However, there is a point at which the frequency of steroid use in a joint becomes unreasonable and destructive. In such cases, with continued progression of joint disease, eventual retirement of the animal from competition or change in its activity may become necessary, rather than increasing the number of joint injections to a more potentially adverse frequency. Your veterinarian will help you make this decision.

Overall, joint injections are safe to the horse when administered by a conscientious practicing veterinarian. Their overall negative effects on joint cartilage are insignificant when they are properly administered at safe intervals. Their anti-inflammatory effect on the joint may persist for many months or longer depending on the underlying stage of joint disease. The horse will be able to perform comfortably and to its ability with judicious use of joint therapies. It may be unfair and inhumane to continue to expect your horse to perform comfortably and successfully without therapy when there is degenerative joint disease. For this reason, if one insists on the exclusion of joint injection for his/her horse, it becomes necessary to manage the condition using the available oral, IM, and IV medications. These therapies are less likely to provide significant relief from degenerative joint disease, as they are best used as "preventive" medications and not as "therapeutic" medications. Without specific joint injection therapy, persistent pain necessitates the horse's retirement and purchase of another if competition is still a goal of the rider.

SHOCK-WAVE THERAPY

A recent advance in the treatment of pain associated with lameness in the horse is the introduction of extracorporeal shock-wave therapy. In this treatment, localized acoustic shock waves are conducted from a hand-held probe to the horse's limb where the pain exists. How this works is as yet undefined. It is believed to produce analgesia (pain relief). At this time, there is believed to be little, if any, anti-inflammatory effect of this treatment. As such, this treatment could be somewhat dangerous to a horse if an accurate diagnosis is not made before treatment. Providing pain relief when there is potential for a catastrophic injury could be a significant concern. Nonetheless, this therapy can be effectively used when a specific diagnosis is made. Foot pain, bruising, navicular disease, mild tendonitis, mild desmitis, and conditions that would be unlikely to progress or cause a catastrophic injury could be and have been successfully addressed with this treatment.

As our understanding of shock-wave therapy and its effects progresses, we will be better equipped to utilize its benefits and minimize the potential for complications.

CHAPTER 9

Common Conditions and Their Prevention

GASTROINTESTINAL CONDITIONS

The most common equine gastrointestinal condition is "colic." This term should not be confused with a specific diagnosis. Colic simply means abdominal pain. As this term does not imply a specific diagnosis, anything that causes abdominal pain causes colic. The possible causes are numerous, ranging from simple gas distension to an impaction of the large intestine to a complete twist of the intestine. Other conditions may also cause colic, such as pregnancy and labor, gastrointestinal ulcers, and infection of the abdominal cavity (peritonitis), among others.

To help prevent colic, it is impor-

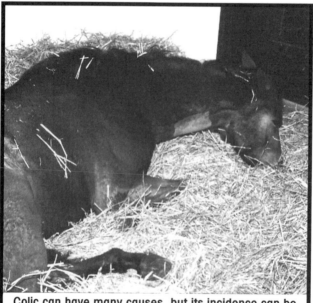

Colic can have many causes, but its incidence can be reduced with preventive measures.

tant to practice preventive medicine. Regular deworming is important to help control gastrointestinal damage and dysfunction associated with parasites. Parasites are a major predisposing factor in all types of colic. Horses in strenuous and regular exercise may experience a high rate of gastrointestinal ulceration. Not all of these horses have clinical disease associated with these ulcers. Gastroscopic examination is helpful in cases of poor appetite, slow eating, and inability to maintain good weight and hair coat. Horses with ulcers may benefit from oral anti-ulcer medications

> ## AT A GLANCE
>
> • Practicing preventive care can help minimize the incidence of conditions such as colic and laminitis.
>
> • Osteoarthritis is typically a chronic but manageable condition.
>
> • Keeping a horse clean and dry can prevent certain coat and skin problems.

such as omeprazole of ranitidine. Other medications administered such as oral antacids and oral cimetidine have less clinical utility against clinically significant ulceration in performance horses.

Providing high-quality feeds and nutrition will also help minimize the likelihood of colic. Changes in feed may also be a significant predisposing factor in various types of colic. For this reason, feeding-program changes should be gradual as described in the chapter on nutrition.

Regular dental care is also important in helping to prevent colic. This care minimizes problems associated with poor dentition such as poor mastication of feed and inability to eat due to dental or oral pain. All things considered, one should not be under the impression that good management precludes colic episodes. Often the specific cause of the colic (such as the cause of an impaction, the cause of a gas colic, the cause of an intestinal twist) remains unclear.

RESPIRATORY CONDITIONS

Conditions that affect the respiratory system may dramatically affect a horse's ability to perform or exercise. For this reason, it is important to maintain respiratory system health and function. Horses should be vaccinated against respiratory pathogens to protect them during periods of likely exposure. Viral respiratory infections may predispose horses to bacterial pneumonia by suppressing normal respiratory epithelial function and respiratory tract immune defenses. Many, if not most, bacterial pneumonias probably begin with a viral respiratory infection; therefore, vaccination is also important in preventing pneumonia in the horse.

The equine influenza vaccine is important to administer to horses regularly encountering other horses. The administration of rhinopneumonitis vaccine (EHV-I and -IV) may be worthwhile. Strangles vaccination may be considered on an individual basis, but it is generally unnecessary for adult horses in competition. Another means of preventing respiratory illness is minimizing the exposure to respiratory irritants and allergens. This means designing a barn for maximal ventilation, use of appropriate low-dust hays, and feeding methods that minimize exposure and inhalation of dust and maximize time outside of the barn. The feeding of round bales should be discouraged because they are associated with higher incidences of colic and botulism. Horses that are stabled for longer periods and in poorly ventilated and managed barns are much more likely to develop lower airway inflammation, bronchiolitis, and chronic obstructive pulmonary disease (COPD or "heaves").

MUSCULAR CONDITIONS

Most muscular conditions involve some predisposing event or exercise that results in the syndrome of "tying-up." During this condition, severe muscle damage may occur, and pigment released from muscle into the blood may cause acute renal failure that, if not successfully treated, can lead to death. Treatment is often intensive and expensive. The best way to help prevent this syndrome is to warm up your horse before the exercise.

Climate extremes may also predispose a horse to tying-up. If a horse is to be expected to perform, compete, or exercise in any extreme of climate, the horse should be acclimated to the new environment for several days or weeks before the event. Assurance of adequate fitness for the expected level of exercise will also minimize the likelihood of tying-up.

Many veterinarians supplement horses with chronic muscular problems with vitamin E and selenium. Performance horses appear to benefit from some vitamin E to their diet. However, many horses that receive selenium supplementation may not benefit from it, as they are not living in selenium-deficient areas. Evaluation of selenium levels in the diet would be warranted before supplementation since oversupplementation causes poor hoof, mane, and tail growth and condition.

Certain heritable conditions such as HYPP and glycogen storage diseases are associated with severe exercise intolerance and muscle damage with a clinical appearance of tying-up. These conditions may be manageable if the disease is not severe in the affected animal. For HYPP, this means generally that those horses that are heterozygous for the two alleles of inheritance (one normal/one affected) may be manageable with low-potassium feeds and hays, medication using acetazolamide, and other practices such as feeding molasses or sweet feed to manage episodes of paralysis. Horses that are homozygous for the two alleles (one affected/ one affected) are much less likely to be capable of exercise in response to the typical methods of management. Horses affected with glycogen storage diseases require dietary changes such as extra fat and fewer carbohydrates. Adequate preparation for the exercise or event is necessary.

SKELETAL CONDITIONS

Many skeletal conditions are associated with degenerative joint disease (osteoarthritis), a common problem in performance horses. Some horses may have problems from a young age when inappropriate formation of joint cartilage led to the production of a joint fragment known as an osteochondral fragment (OCD). Osteoarthritis is typically a chronic condition that is manageable by many of the therapies suggested in this book. Management often is successful for many years, but occasionally the condition advances to an extent at which the frequency of joint injections, cost of medications, and/or the success of the treatments become inadequate to provide sufficient soundness for continued competition. In such a situation, retirement from that competition may be necessary. However, many of those types of horses make the best school horses for younger and more inexperienced riders, who benefit from the seasoned horses' experience and ease of riding.

Other skeletal conditions that can occur may affect the "soft tissue" connections of the muscle and bone: the tendons and ligaments. Acute or chronic injuries to these structures are common and painful. They often require significant time to heal. If they can heal, the structure may not be as strong as it once was. Common injuries of this type include "bowed tendons" of the superficial and deep flexor tendons and injuries to the suspensory ligament.

Acute fracture of any bones, particularly in the leg, is a possibility and a concern for horses engaged in nearly any type of competition. In years past, such fractures usually meant no alternative other than humane destruction of the animal. However, great advances have been made in management and repair of limb fractures in the horse. A qualified veterinarian should evaluate each case to determine whether an injury warrants surgery or another treatment option.

FOOT CONDITIONS

Foot problems and conditions are minimized by regular foot care. Hoof trimming should be considered every four to eight weeks, depending on the rate of growth and presence of foot problems. Normal hoof growth for an adult is about 0.25 to 0.35 inches per month. Some horses, such as Thoroughbreds, may have very flat and thin soles. Without regular shoeing, such horses may exhibit intermittent or chronic foot soreness and lameness. Horses should be trimmed according to their individual conformation and not based on what the "picture of the correct foot" might be. A horse should be trimmed so its feet land flat, and individual differences in conformation might require slightly different trimming to allow the foot to land flat. Horses should not be allowed to grow too long in the toe of the hoof or to grow underneath the foot from the bulbs of the heel. Appropriate foot length allows proper orientation of the foot below the axis of the leg, and thus good support of the limb during motion and exercise.

Navicular disease affects the navicular bone in the heel. The condition typically affects both front feet, causing intermittently mild to severe lameness. The presentation may be that of only unilateral lameness. However, the diagnosis is made by appropriate lameness examination with nerve blocks that indicate pain in the heel. Typically, after one side is blocked, the horse becomes lamer or noticeably lame in the opposite front foot. The cause of navicular disease is poorly understood. This becomes obvious when one is exposed to the various ideas and opinions that pertain to its management and treatment. There are numerous purported approaches to the treatment of this disease, and no one approach seems to be uniformly successful. Anti-inflammatory therapy and shoeing changes are typically advocated.

The role of the drug isoxsuprine in the treatment of this disease appears to be severely overstated because the horse's ability to absorb this drug in the intestine after oral administration is poor at best (about two percent of the amount given orally). Other medications have been attempted with limited success and no real scientific support of their efficacy. Shoeing changes have typically involved putting a pad beneath the shoe. Often these pads are "wedge pads" that elevate the heel. Shoeing changes, in my experience, are best approached from a trial-and-error basis.

Ultimately, navicular disease may become severe enough to consider euthanasia or a salvage procedure known as a neurectomy. A neurectomy is the removal of a segment of the nerve supplying the navicular area of the foot. It is a salvage procedure because it can lead to catastrophic rupture of the deep flexor tendon. For this reason, it may be advisable not to ride such horses once this procedure has been performed.

Laminitis is another major condition affecting the foot. The primary problem in the case of laminitis is the development of inflammation and poor blood supply to the area where the hard hoof wall of the foot attaches to the bone in the foot called the coffin bone (or P3). When this occurs, the horse's weight may act as a force that tears the hoof wall away from the coffin bone (rotation) or causes the coronary band to separate and push the entire bone downward and through the sole of the foot (sinking). This condition is extremely painful in all of its stages. Medical management and frog support or more elaborate changes in the shoeing techniques and materials used may provide adequate support to allow recovery from the bout of laminitis. However, any rotation or sinking that has occurred may be difficult or impossible to correct. Typically horses that have experienced one episode of laminitis are at a higher risk of having another episode of acute pain and further progression of the rotation and/or sinking.

As is the case of navicular disease, the overall understanding of this disease is poor. As such, many therapies are used to treat it, some with reported success (either theoretically or clinically justified). Major aspects of therapy include analgesics and anti-inflammatory drugs (excluding steroids — as they have been associated with the development of laminitis) and foot support, either on the foot itself or by changing the footing of a stall to sand. Treatment of the underlying diseases or conditions is necessary.

Underlying diseases (such as diarrhea, severe pneumonias, and severe uterine infections) that may be associated with the development of laminitis must be treated. Newer approaches to therapy have included topical nitroglycerin paste and advanced and innovative shoeing techniques. Hoof wall resection has been advocated in the treatment of laminitis to allow for "realignment." This is a heroic procedure and is often extremely painful to the animal. Significant caution should be exercised before pursuing any heroic measures for this condition. This means weighing the *realistic* likelihood for success and what the consideration of success is (pasture sound versus an animal that is capable of performing) against cost of treatment and humane considerations (amount of pain that is reasonable to expect the horse to have to go through and/or live with).

From the management aspect of hoof care, it is advisable to clean and pick the soles of the horse's feet daily or more often. Horses should be provided with adequate footing for safety and dryness to prevent thrush or other infectious and destructive conditions of the hoof wall. Black walnut shavings should never be used as they are associated with the development of laminitis. Hoof-wall dressings and paints and sole paints may

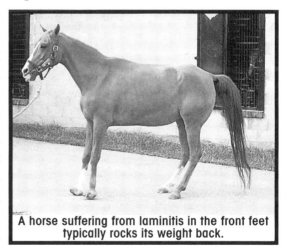

A horse suffering from laminitis in the front feet typically rocks its weight back.

provide protection and/or hardening of the foot. They should not be overused.

An owner or trainer should decide on the selection of a farrier based on skill, availability, personality, willingness to work with clients and teach them about his role, and ability to work well with the veterinarian. Many cases of foot problems and shoeing require a joint effort and cooperation between the farrier and the veterinarian.

NERVOUS SYSTEM CONDITIONS

Fortunately, nervous system conditions are relatively uncommon in horses, but they are more common in this species than in many other species. Measures to prevent development of nervous system conditions are relatively undefined. Certain conditions such as "wobbler syndrome" may be associated with rapid growth and dietary imbalances of certain nutrients. This condition is associated with compression of the spinal cord by the vertebrae in the neck. This typically causes loss of coordination of the hind legs and sometimes of the forelegs as well. The disease is highly suspect in young (two- to three-year-old) horses that are growing fast and have the abnormal coordination described. There could be a genetic component to the development of this syndrome. Therefore, maintaining a reasonable growth rate and a good diet, and avoiding breedings that have produced wobblers in the past may be the limit to what can be realistically done to try and prevent wobbler syndrome.

Equine protozoal myeloencephalitis is the other major nervous system disease that is the primary alternative diagnosis to wobbler syndrome for horses that show loss of coordination of the hind limbs and/or the forelimbs without any other signs. EPM cannot be definitively diagnosed in a live horse. Despite the existence of diagnostic tests for this disease, the tests are fraught with complexities that hamper their interpretation and

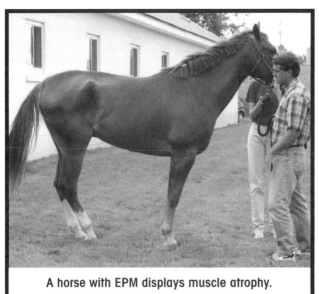

A horse with EPM displays muscle atrophy.

cannot be relied on alone as definite indicators of the disease state. Prevention of EPM should focus on preventing opossums and other known hosts access to feed sources and discouraging their presence on pasture. Opossums pass the stage of the parasite that is apparently ingested by horses and causes disease in a small percentage of those exposed to the parasite. Although the impression of the incidence of EPM might be much greater, the estimated rate of disease is well less than 1 percent of the horse population despite exposure rates to all horses of 50 percent to nearly 90 percent.

Nervous system disorders associated with previous respiratory infection, hind limb loss of coordination, and loss of ability to control the bladder may be associated with equine herpesvirus I infection. Trauma is a common cause for nervous system conditions. Clinical signs depend on the area of the nervous system affected. Other conditions might include otitis media/interna (middle and inner ear disease) and a number of other somewhat less common conditions.

SKIN, COAT, AND MANE AND TAIL CONDITIONS

"Rain rot" (*Dermatophilus congolensis*) is an infectious condition of the skin and is often seen in horses that have been exposed excessively to rain or wet conditions. The changes in the coat occur along the back and over the croup. It causes black crusting lesions that are easily removed from the skin. The condition is best managed by regular grooming and by avoidance of wet conditions. In severe cases, antibiotic therapy may be warranted.

Dermatophytosis (ringworm) is caused by a fungal infection of the skin. It is highly contagious and can be transmitted to a human. The lesions are circular in appearance and cause hair loss over the affected areas. Hair can usually be plucked from the affected site easily. Preventing spread of the infection in the barn requires individual use of grooming implements and tack for the affected horse only. Most cases will resolve spontaneously, but treatment usually minimizes the spread of the condition. Treatment may not significantly shorten the course of the infection. Topical fungal washes or oral griseofulvin are commonly used for treatment. Many practitioners use a fungicide called captan because it is relatively inexpensive and appears to be effective. Caution should be exercised in the use of this or other fungicidal powders as they are potentially toxic to both the horse and humans.

External parasites are somewhat uncommon in horses. Problems associated with external parasites may be minimized by regular and complete deworming, minimizing exposure to external parasites, and good care of the skin, coat and mane, and tail. Good skin and coat care are best provided by regular brushing. Shampooing of the coat is advisable with a shampoo strong enough to remove dirt but mild enough to allow the skin and hair's natural oils to remain. Shampooing too frequently will remove these oils. Thorough rinsing of soap from the coat will also help the coat retain natural oils. Protein-based hair conditioners may be used to coat the hair shaft.

Chronic illness may produce a poor coat by decreasing the production of skin oils. Good nutrition is part of this consideration. Excess or inadequate levels of a nutrient, vitamin A deficiency or excess, protein deficiency, or deficiency in the essential fatty acid linoleic acid may cause poor coat and skin condition. Adding one to two ounces of corn, safflower, or soy oil is frequently used to provide luster to a coat.

CARDIOVASCULAR CONDITIONS

Cardiovascular problems, which are relatively uncommon, may cause exercise intolerance in performance horses. Some conditions may be associated with the timing and rate of the heartbeat. These abnormalities in rhythm may lead to poor performance. However, a common "physiologic arrhythmia" (an arrhythmia that occurs due to the different physiology of the horse) is called second-degree AV block. This arrhythmia is most often associated with intense nerve input that dampens or slows the normal resting heart rate in a horse. It produces a regular heart rhythm with an occasional "dropped beat." It is most often not associated with any heart problem and as such has no implications on performance. It disappears when the horse is stimulated or excited so that the normal dampening effect of the vagus nerve is overrun by the sympathetic nervous drive on the heart (the fight-or-flight response). Other arrhythmias that occur in the horse with relative infrequency may be related to exercise intolerance and poor performance. Atrial fibrillation is one of the more common arrhythmias recognized, but others are possible.

Other conditions that may affect the performance and overall health of the horse are cardiac murmurs associated with abnormal blood flow through a heart valve. Heart murmurs may be significant findings in the horse, but the severity varies. As there are "physiologic arrhythmias" in the horse, so too are there "physiologic flow murmurs" that are not associated with any abnormal or pathologic condition in the equine heart, but are instead associated with normal blood flow in the equine heart due to its size and the size of the vessels into which the blood flows. Mild murmurs associated with an abnormal blood flow or abnormal heart chamber pressures may cause little or no immediate significance to a horse. Indeed, many horses with only mild incidence of abnormal blood flow and pressure changes due to a pathologic murmur may never experience significant clinical effect and may die of old age long before the murmur becomes symptomatic. However, murmurs associated with larger amounts of abnormal blood flow and pressure changes in the heart may cause exercise intolerance and reduced performance in horses used for competition and exercise.

In reality, no specific management or therapies can prevent this type of disease. The best approach is to keep your horse healthy and well-vaccinated and dewormed. A routine physical examination should be performed at least yearly. During such an examination, your veterinarian will listen to the heart for normal rhythms and murmurs. If an arrhythmia or a murmur is detected, your veterinarian should be able to help you decide whether it is "physiologic" (not associated with a problem) or "pathologic" (associated with an abnormality). If there is any question about the finding, consultation with a certified expert can provide answers and/or the necessary diagnostic equipment to outline specifically the cause of the arrhythmia or the murmur. Again, not all arrhythmias and murmurs are pathologic, and in performance horses "physiologic" arrhythmias and murmurs are very common.

ANTIMICROBIAL USE IN HORSES/ IMMUNOTHERAPY
Indications

Antimicrobial drugs (antibiotics) are commonly administered to horses for numerous conditions or reasons. Antimicrobial use in the horse has extended beyond veterinary use to include common administration by owners and trainers, with or without veterinary consultation. Although the wider availability of antibiotic medications has minimized the cost of treatments and allowed for early treatment of potentially significant conditions, veterinary consultation should always be sought prior to administration. Indeed, in some areas, antibiotics are likely being misused.

Veterinary consultation is not recommended for the benefit of veterinarians. Consideration of the need for antibiotics, the type of antibiotic, the potential side effects, cost, dosage, and potential for interaction with other medications are all issues that a veterinarian considers before deciding to administer an antibiotic. Cavalier administration of any available antibiotic may cause significant problems, depending on the horse and the condition being addressed. Furthermore, viral infectious processes may not require antibiotic administration at all since viruses are insensitive to conventional antibiotic therapy. The risks of side effects such as antibiotic-induced diarrhea and other drug-specific adverse effects are important to consider. Finally, administration of an available antibiotic may not be appropriate for the organism causing the infection. Therefore, good working knowledge of the common organisms associated with various infections and the spectrums of activity of the antibiotics available are important to maximize the likelihood that the selected antibiotic will eliminate the infection. Finally, the duration of antibiotic treatment is a necessary consideration, as antibiotic therapy that is discontinued too early will be unsuccessful. This also requires a working understanding of the characteristics of each antibiotic and of the infectious process that is being treated. These decisions are best addressed through veterinary consultation.

Misuse of antibiotics by underdosing or by providing an inadequate duration of therapy allows for the development and perpetuation of organism resistance. With continued use of this nature, bacteria will continue to develop mechanisms by which they can escape the activity and effects of previously effective antibiotics. Veterinary consultation will help minimize this effect and is highly recommendable.

Immunotherapy

The use of immunotherapy has increased over the past few years. This therapy is directed at placing the immune system on "stand by" for the potential exposure to infective and disease-causing organisms or to "boost" the function of the immune system against a pathogen that is affecting the horse. The most common products used for this type of therapy include Eq-Stim®, Equimune IV®, and oral levamisole. These therapies have received some positive testimonials, but the existence of specific scientific information supporting their use is limited. There have been infrequent reports of a granulomatous pneumonia that has been associated with the administration of an intravenously administered product. Therefore, although there may be certain instances when such type of therapy could be helpful, the use of such products should be thoroughly discussed with a veterinarian.

CHAPTER 10

Preventive Medicine in Aging Horses and Horses with Common Chronic Conditions

AGING HORSES

To maximize an aging horse's quality and length of life, the owner often needs to address health considerations. Aging horses commonly have problems with their teeth and maintaining weight. Older broodmares may become more difficult to get bred. Horses that are used for performance should not be expected to compete at the same level as before. The incidence of pituitary tumors becomes increasingly common in aging horses. These tumors appear to be very common in older horses and often add to the debilitation of aging by causing excessive drinking and urinating, long hair coats that shed out poorly, chronic infections, poor body condition, and the possibility of laminitis. Aging and chronic conditions associated with aging, such as osteoarthritis, will eventually lead to weakened performance. Retirement or a change to a less intensive occupation eventually becomes warranted.

ESOPHAGEAL DISORDERS

Disorders of the esophagus, such as esophageal diverticulum or esophageal strictures, may cause chronic problems during eating. Such horses are predisposed to develop esophageal obstruction, or "choke." Horses diagnosed with such problems will require special attention to feeding and types of feed offered. Less serious cases will require that the horse receive only soft, green hay or grasses and easily masti- cated and swallowed feeds for a finite period. More severe cases may require complete avoid- ance of hay, only limited access to grasses, and the feeding of "slurries" or "soups" made from complete pelleted or extruded feeds. Continued problems with "choke" may require even more intensive therapies. If weight loss associated with this condi-

> ## AT A GLANCE
>
> • Some older horses have special dietary needs.
>
> • Aging horses commonly have problems with their teeth and maintaining weight.
>
> • Euthanasia should be considered when a horse is suffering and the prognosis for recovery is poor.

tion becomes severe, euthanasia may become a consideration.

PITUITARY ADENOMA (CUSHING'S SYNDROME)

Pituitary adenoma is a tumor that becomes increasingly common with age in horses. The clinical signs of this tumor include excess drinking and urination, long poor-quality hair coat, weak pendulous abdomen, muscle loss along the back, repetitive infections of the skin and other body systems, and chronic laminitis. The tumor causes excess production of adrenocorticotropic hormone (ACTH) and associated pro- teins and hormones. This condition can often be diagnosed on characteristic clinical signs alone. However, confirming the diagnosis is recommended. The typical confirmation in- cludes endocrine function testing using an ACTH stimulation test or a dexamethasone suppression test. Confirmatory testing is necessary to treat the condition. Medical manage- ment of the disease involves administering a dopamine agonist (pergolide or bromocriptine) or a serotonin antago- nist (cyproheptadine). Treatment appears to be successful at improving clinical signs associated with the condition. Pergolide is often reported to be most effective, but it is also the most expensive. Cyproheptadine has been reported to produce good rates of success, while the expense is significantly less. Horses with this condition must receive excellent access to water, appropriate diets, dental care, deworming, and hoof care, as horses with this tumor are more susceptible to associated problems. Laminitis can become difficult to manage, and overfeeding of hay and/or grain must be strictly avoided.

CHRONIC OBSTRUCTIVE PULMONARY DISEASE (HEAVES)

As is the case for other chronic conditions, "heaves" is not curable, but it can be managed with good feeding practices and minimizing exposure to airway irritants and/or allergens. This condition is caused by hyper-responsiveness of the equine airway to dusts, molds, and fungi in the horse's environment. These irritants constrict the smooth muscle lining the small airways and cause excess production of mucus and recruitment of inflammatory cells and products. These factors together restrict normal respiration and gas exchange normally performed by the lung. This increases respiratory effort and rate and often produces a chronic cough. There may be episodes of severe distress with nostril flare and heavy abdominal breathing. This condition is analogous to asthma in people.

Not all horses are so severely affected that they exhibit the obvious clinical signs described above. Indeed, there appear to be degrees of severity for conditions like this that affect the horse's lungs. Less severe manifestations can include a chronic, dry cough that may be worse during exercise, mild to moderate exercise intolerance, or inability to perform to full potential. Such horses may be affected with less severe airway irritation, chronic inflammation, and bronchiolitis.

The management for COPD and less severe lower respiratory inflammatory conditions such as bronchiolitis are similar. Minimize the amount of exposure to dusts, molds, and fungi. This means feeding of low-dust feeds and hay in manners that minimize the inhalation of particles from the food source; maximizing the amount of time outside of an enclosure such as a barn, if necessary; feeding water-soaked hay and/or grains/pellets; turning out horses while sweeping the barn and mucking stalls; etc. It is important that horses with conditions such as COPD are well-vaccinated and dewormed in order to maximize health and prevent secondary bacterial infections that might be more common in horses with this condition.

Medical management of COPD and lower airway inflammation should be administered during "episodes" associated with worsening of clinical signs. Acute treatment for such episodes often involves the administration of an oral bronchodilating agent such as clenbuterol and a fast-acting steroid. Continuing therapy for a few days with both medications is often advised, with the steroids being tapered off. Maintenance therapy has often been advocated by the daily administration of oral prednisolone. The use of oral steroid therapy and oral bronchodilator therapy should be chosen carefully. Recent evidence indicates that orally administered prednisone (as opposed to prednisolone) and oral albuterol (a bronchodilator) are poorly absorbed by the horse. Therefore, they are less likely to have significant clinical effect. The more appropriate oral medications might therefore be clenbuterol (Ventipulmin®️ syrup) and prednisolone. Short-term steroid therapy using dexamethasone powder (Azium®️) has also been effective in helping control acute exacerbation of clinical signs. Inhalant medications such as albuterol (Torpex®️) and steroids are becoming increasingly available and are likely to be very helpful in management of this condition.

AGE-RELATED GASTROINTESTINAL DIGESTIVE INEFFICIENCY

As has already been discussed, some horses develop difficulty in maintaining weight as they age. A reasonable approach to this problem begins with assuring good health care for older horses. This requires special attention to controlling intestinal parasites, maintaining good dental care and health, and maintaining other aspects of health care to minimize the effects of disease on the older horse. Regular deworming and dental care will help assure that the older horse can masticate and swallow comfortably and effectively, and that the calories and nutrients that are swallowed do not have to be shared with intestinal parasites.

Some horses, despite excellent health care, continue to have difficulty maintaining weight as they age. Very old horses may have few or no teeth left for mastication of hay and grains. Such horses will probably require complete pelleted or extruded feeds that can be offered as a food "slurry" or "soup." Horses that have some dentition left but that are still only poorly maintaining their body weight may also benefit from a more digestible formulation for older horses. Hay fed to these horses should be high quality, soft, and green. Horses that continue to have difficulty in maintaining weight should be thoroughly evaluated by a veterinarian for dental or other oral problems and possible conditions that might lead to an inability to maintain weight.

LAMINITIS

Maintaining health and comfort of horses that have been diagnosed with laminitis can be a large undertaking, but it is imperative in order to maximize the overall quality of life for these animals. Horses with chronic laminitis or those that have been previously diagnosed with laminitis are at risk of recurrence. For such horse, high-quality preventive medicine is helpful to minimize the likelihood of the development of illness. Illness of any kind in these horses could easily lead to recurrence of laminitis. Good vaccination and deworming are important considerations. Nutrition is an important component of preventive care of these horses. Overfeeding is a risk for horses previously diagnosed with laminitis. Horses that are overweight must be placed on diets to minimize unnecessary stress and forces on the affected feet. Underlying health problems should be addressed appropriately to control these risk factors for recurrence of laminitis.

Regular foot care is imperative. Most horses with laminitis probably do better in shoes. Unshod horses might be more prone to foot pain and inflammation associated with laminitis. Trimming is usually performed to minimize the length of toe and/or the pull of the deep flexor tendon on the coffin bone. For some cases, good trimming also helps "reorient" the coffin bone to a more normal position relative to the hoof wall. Shoeing such horses often becomes trial and error to find the most comfortable shoes and orientation of the foot. Commonly used shoes include heart bar shoes, bar shoes, shoes with wedge pads, and regular shoes. Depending on the severity of the laminitis, the degree of rotation, the amount of coffin bone sinking, and time since the last episode of pain associated with laminitis, horses might respond to the above options differently. Horses undergoing painful episodes of laminitis have also responded to specially made plastic glue-on or taped-on shoes with rubber-like cushions that conform to the sole and elevate the heel.

Medical therapy may be necessary intermittently for periods of increased pain associated with laminitis. Typical treatments used are the same in acute first-time laminitis. Most medical therapy is directed at providing analgesia and decreasing inflammation. Phenylbutazone, flunixin meglumine (Banamine®), and ketoprofen are often used for this purpose. Extended use of these NSAIDs may be associated with intestinal ulceration and kidney dysfunction. For this reason extended treatment using high doses of these medications should be avoided or carefully administered. Addition of anti-ulcer medications such as omeprazole or ranitidine may be worthwhile considerations. Phenylbutazone appears to be the most dangerous with respect to these side effects; flunixin meglumine, less so but still of significant concern. Ketoprofen may be least ulcerogenic but still should be used judiciously. It is more expensive and is administered by injection.

A final word on laminitis is warranted. Although emotional attachment may play a large role in your desire as an owner to continue therapy and attempt to control this condition, I urge you to consider and openly discuss with your veterinarian the need and indeed the humanity of a decision to elect for euthanasia in horses exhibiting chronic pain associated with laminitis. Making such a decision when your horse is in this condition is difficult. However, I would caution the owner of a seriously laminitic horse against unreal expectations of comfort and complete recovery for horses whose coffin bones are severely rotated or sinking. Although it is possible for some horses that appear to be severely affected to recover over time, the odds tend not to be in favor of recovery of severely rotated or sinking horses. Indeed, even if recovery is a possibility, I urge you to ask yourself and discuss with your veterinarian and farrier what price you are willing to impose on the horse and how much pain you feel it should have to endure in order to have what may be a limited chance of a comfortable existence.

CHRONIC MUSCULOSKELETAL DISEASES (ARTHRITIS, ETC.)

Horses with chronic musculoskeletal disorders may benefit from periodic administration of analgesic medications such as NSAIDs to help control pain when it is at its worst. Conditions such as osteoarthritis (degenerative joint disease) may also benefit from regular administration of oral joint supplements containing chondroitin sulfates and glucosamine, administration of IV hyaluronic acid preparations (Legend®), IM administration of polysulfated glycosaminoglycans (Adequan IM®), and other supportive therapies or combinations of these.

Intra-articular administrations (injections into the affected joint) of hyaluronic acid and/or polysulfated glycosaminoglycans may be more effective in helping to protect and restore health to joint cartilage. Intra-articular steroid therapy is often useful to remove acute or chronic inflammation of an affected joint, to provide rapid pain relief, and to support joint health and function further when it is mixed with hyaluronic acid. If frequent repetitive use of intra-articular steroid therapy becomes necessary to maintain athletic performance, reduction in the level or intensity of the exercise or competition or retirement from competition should be seriously considered. Breeding of genetically adequate animals is also a viable alternative when this point is reached.

Management considerations for horses with chronic musculoskeletal conditions include routine vaccination and deworming, good nutrition that prevents the development of obesity, good footing in all areas where such horses are kept or have access, regular monitoring for exacerbations of the conditions, and the availability of appropriate medical therapy when needed for these conditions.

CHAPTER 11

Housing, Bedding, and Fencing

Stabling, pasturing, bedding, and other aspects of a horse's living environment have major implications on the potential for health problems.

With the domestication of horses, we have imposed the need to house large numbers of animals in one or a group of barns or other facilities that permit easier care while minimizing our discomfort and exposure to the elements. While helpful for the caretaker, this has brought new problems and health concerns for horses in this situation. Two major problems with stabling horses in barns are generally poor ventilation and a high concentration of animals for disease communication. A barn intended to stable horses should be designed with ventilation in mind. At least eight complete air

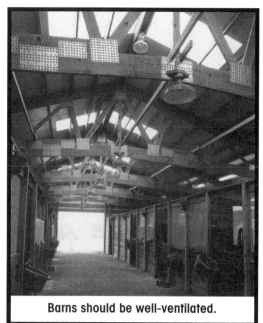

Barns should be well-ventilated.

changes should take place each hour in a stable if good-quality bedding and hay are used. (The volume of air equal to the volume of the barn enters the barn and leaves it eight times per hour with good ventilation.) This is necessary to help minimize dissemination of aerosol-spread diseases and to minimize exposure to air irritants and allergens. Barns need not be heated for horses to be comfortable. In fact, most horses thrive in cold weather as long as they are kept dry and out of direct wind. Heating barns and closing their doors to keep in the warmth benefit people working in such barns

AT A GLANCE

• Well-ventilated barns help minimize the spread of certain diseases, irritants, and allergens.

• Regular care minimizes foot problems and conditions.

• Horses should receive dental examinations once or twice a year.

• An important component of practicing preventive medicine and care for your horse(s) includes maintaining complete and accurate health records.

but are less than ideal for the horses. Such practices increase humidity within the barn. A humid environment further adds to the growth of bacteria and mold. Personnel in show barns often blanket horses and heat barns during the cold months in order to maintain short-hair coats on the horses. Again, this is not ideal for the health of the horse but appears to be necessary by today's show standards. If blanketing is practiced, care should be taken not to blanket so heavily that the horse(s) is caused to sweat.

Barn flooring should be made of good footing, and the aisle ways and stall floors should allow efficient cleaning. Many times dirt floors are preferable to concrete or blacktop flooring, but they allow bacteria to grow and hold moisture from urine and other fluids. An alternative to these flooring ideas in stalls is placement of stall mats. Mats may become damp and musty on the underside; therefore, as for dirt floors, it is advisable to clean and dry the mats routinely.

Horses may be bedded on numerous types of material. Commonly used materials include straw, shavings, and sawdust. All bedding material should be inspected for significant amounts of dust, mold, and insects or other parasites such as chiggers. Less commonly used bedding types include newspaper, peat, and hay.

Muck piles should be distant from the barn and horses to minimize exposure to parasites and insects that live in or are attracted to them.

Regular manure and bedding removal is important. Composting may also be a practical way to control manure and waste removal from stalls.

Horses living solely on pasture should have access to a "run-in shed" or some other shelter to protect them from direct wind and rain.

Another consideration for preventing injuries and problems with horses is fencing. A number of types of fencing are now available for livestock and horses. However, generally speaking, fencing that is appropriate for cattle or other animals including barbed-wire fencing and high-tensile wire may not be good choices for horses. Barbed wire and high-tensile wire fencing tend to cause severe lacerations in horses that run into it or that simply get a leg caught. Vinyl post-and-rail fencing, wood post-and-rail fencing, and wood split-rail fencing tend to be sturdier and not to lead to such severe cuts and injuries. However, these types of fencing are significantly more expensive and are subject to wood chewing and cribbing. Vinyl fencing may melt under high temperatures generated by a fire or other intense heat source.

Electric fences have been used with some success. However, if a horse is spooked, it can easily run through this type of fencing. The premise to electric fencing is that the horses develop an aversion to the fence after having been shocked. However, many owners prefer the peace of mind of sturdier fencing more capable of withstanding a horse's impact and preventing its escape onto nearby roads or other dangerous areas. Some people have combined electric fencing with other types of fencing to maximize the safety and protection of otherwise less ideal fencing, while minimizing expense.

Another type of fencing that is less expensive and appears to be very strong and very safe is vinyl-tape fencing. This fencing is made of high-tensile wire covered with vinyl stripping. Because it is covered, it loses its tendency to cause cuts on impact. Furthermore, it can stretch a great distance even under the severe impact of animals the size of horses. A final consideration in fencing is inevitably its appearance. Much of the wood fencing and the vinyl-post and rail fencings tend to be most attractive. However, the newer vinyl-tape fencing comes in a number of widths, and the widest size mimics the appearance of regular vinyl post-and-rail fencing while still having the characteristics of the tape fencing and the persistence of a wire, even if all of the vinyl were to melt from a fire, at a relatively reduced expense.

SOME PRINCIPLES OF HOOF CARE

Regular care minimizes foot problems and conditions. Hoof trimming should be considered every four to eight weeks depending on the rate of growth and presence of foot problems. Normal hoof growth for an adult is about 0.25 to 0.35 inches per month. Some horses, such as Thoroughbreds, may have very flat and thin soles. Without regular shoeing, such horses may exhibit intermittent or chronic foot soreness and lameness. Horses should be trimmed according to their

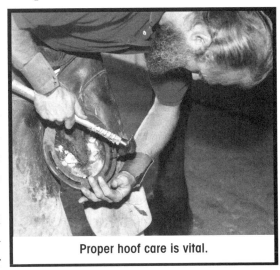

Proper hoof care is vital.

individual conformation and not based on what the "picture of the correct foot" might be. A horse should be trimmed so its foot will land flat, and individual variations in conformation might require slightly different trimming to allow the foot to land flat. The toe of the hoof should not be allowed to grow too long nor should the hoof grow too long underneath from the bulbs of the heel. This is to allow proper orientation of the foot below the axis of the leg and thus good support of the limb during motion and exercise.

DENTAL CARE

Regular dental care is important to help maintain good overall health of a horse. Furthermore, problems associated with teeth or oral pain may prohibit a horse from responding to a bit. Dental care is usually provided by a complete oral examination and regular floating (filing down) of teeth on a yearly or twice-yearly basis. Horse's teeth are continually erupting. Routine floating is needed to control sharp edges formed by chewing and the wear of the teeth due to chewing. Sharp edges typically develop on the outside of the upper dental arcade and on the inside of the lower dental arcade. Horses may also develop points on the occlusal (the chewing surface) surfaces of teeth. These may be found on molars or even pre-molar teeth. Such points should also be floated to prevent malocclusion and pain associated with eating. Horses that have a tooth removed in one arcade will have the opposing tooth grow overly long due to the loss of occlusion and wear on the tooth that is left.

Horses' teeth are constantly erupting (emerging through the gums) as the grinding action wears away the crown surface. Many horses are living much longer lives and are outliving the length of the teeth they have to erupt. When the horse runs out of eruptible tooth, the wear of the teeth continues until there is essentially no tooth left. At this point, mastication and digestion of food become more difficult for the horse. Changes in feed are often necessary. Older horses may also develop "wave mouth," a condition that occurs with unequal wear of the occlusal surface of the teeth. This can also be associated with poor feed mastication and oral pain. It requires good dental care to continue to maximize the use of the remaining teeth.

Trainers and dentists must regularly address wolf teeth. Not all horses have wolf teeth. However, there is the impression that when they are present, wolf teeth (the second pre-molar) must be removed. Although this is common practice, it may be unnecessary.

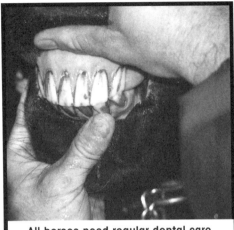

All horses need regular dental care.

Trainers and owners are often concerned about potential discomfort associated with wolf teeth and a bit. However, this is often not a problem, and wolf tooth extraction could be approached reasonably on an "as needed" basis. Nonetheless, many owners and trainers choose to have them extracted before any potential problems might occur.

Dental care should be provided by a qualified individual. There are a number of highly skilled equine dentists and veterinarians with interests and skills in equine dentistry. A little research and "word of mouth" are probably indicated to find a dentist for your horse(s).

HORSES WITH BEHAVIORAL PROBLEMS

Behavioral problems in horses are probably a product of their domestication and our choices of housing for them. Stereotypical behaviors of horses may include stall walking, fence walking, wood chewing, cribbing, self-mutilation. Other behavioral problems that may be learned include kicking, biting, excessive aggression, rearing, bucking, headshaking, and disrespect for a person leading or holding the horse.

Behavioral problems might be minimized by providing adequate environmental stimulation to the horse. This includes adequate turn-out, perhaps with other horses, feeding free-choice hay while in the stall, allowing visual contact with other horses in the barn, and regular interactions with the horse such as grooming, riding, and hand grazing.

Behaviors may be difficult to control once learned. Preventing them might be more successful. Good training and management are imperative to teach a horse, especially a young horse, good manners and to prevent behaviors that are learned because of inadequate discipline and handling.

Behavioral problems can be extremely frustrating to the owner or trainer. Some behaviors are more amenable to control and are more benign in their implications. For instance, cribbing can often be controlled by placement of a cribbing collar or strap. The effect of cribbing on the horse is minimal. Hypertrophy of some neck muscles may be possible with chronic uncontrolled cribbing. Contrary to popular belief, there is no substantial evidence that cribbing leads to an increased incidence of "gas colic." Other stereotypical behaviors may occur out of boredom. Providing a companion goat or other horse or donkey, feeding free-choice hay, and providing other environmental stimulation with toys or other interesting items may help alleviate such behavior.

For persistent problems relating to behavior, a veterinary examination is warranted. On occasion some abnormal behaviors occur out of pain or the anticipation of pain with performance, exercise, or particular motions or situations. A veterinary opinion will help determine whether a medical or orthopedic problem might be causing the behavior. If not, your veterinarian might suggest some further approaches. For chronic behavioral problems that are not responsive to these suggestions, consultation with an equine behavioral specialist/therapist might be the best option.

KEEPING RECORDS ON YOUR HORSE

An important component of practicing preventive medicine and care for your horse(s) includes maintaining complete and accurate records on their health care and their treatment and management practices.

Good health records should include:

- horse's (s') name(s), with names of sire and dam, breed, and registration numbers
- identification: sex, color, markings, tattoos, brands, scars, and weight and height
- foaling date and history
- health history with dates
- vaccinations
- dewormings
- illnesses and injuries
- dental examinations and care administered
- foot care
- physical examinations
- diagnostic tests run: Coggins tests, EVA testing, etc.
- any diagnosed allergies
- feeding program: frequency and amounts, supplements utilized
- performance activity and records
- breeding history and reproductive examinations
- rectal palpations
- vaginal exam
- Caslick's surgeries
- application of artificial lighting
- uterine biopsies and cultures
- dates of estrus
- hormonal therapy
- teasing record
- breeding: method, to whom, by whom
- foaling dates: details of foaling, problems, etc.; growth rate
- boarding history
- owners: names, address, when, and where

CHAPTER 12

Complementary Therapies

Complementary therapy includes therapeutic modalities that are used to augment standard medical therapies. It may also be used as preventive therapy for various conditions and pain or other clinical signs associated with these conditions. Complementary therapies should not be used to take the place of conventional medical practices.

In some instances a lack of response to conventional medical practices leads people to try complementary therapies. In such instances, complementary therapies may be helpful. However, most do not specifically address the underlying problem or disease process. If a conventional medical practice doesn't work, in addition to considering complementary therapies, it is probably prudent for the attending veterinarian to review the diagnosis. A major reason for inadequate or lack of response to therapy is an inaccurate diagnosis.

Examples of complementary therapy recognized by the American Association of Equine Practitioners include acupuncture, chiropractic care, homeopathy, herbology, massage therapy, and physical therapy. Alternative and complementary veterinary medicine approaches to these therapies include veterinary botanical medicine, nutraceutical medicine, and holistic veterinary medicine. The American Association of Equine Practitioners' position is that practitioners of alternative and complementary medicine should have received significant education in the areas practiced.

This often means taking specific courses in the particular complementary therapy practiced and passing an examination of certification in that area.

CHIROPRACTIC CARE

Some veterinarians and other trained individuals use chiropractic care to help address spinal and other related skeletal disorders. The practitioner manipulates the spine to address pain possibly caused by malalignment of vertebrae or other spinal structures. This modality of therapy has received increasing support by veterinarians and laypersons alike. However, as is the case for all complementary therapies, misuse or poor application is unlikely to be helpful and may even be harmful. As is the case for all complementary therapies, this treatment has limits. Chiropractic manipulations should not take the place of

> ## AT A GLANCE
>
> • Complementary therapies should not be used to take the place of conventional medical practices.
>
> • Complementary therapy can be used as a preventive factor for various conditions.
>
> • Chiropractic and acupuncture continue to gain support, and their use is increasing.

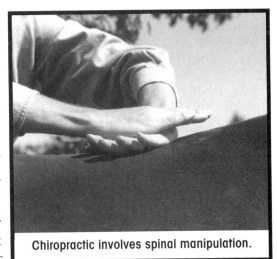

Chiropractic involves spinal manipulation.

conventional therapies and complete lameness examinations. Appropriate case selection and application of chiropractic care are important to maximize its utility, safety, and results. Certified equine chiropractors should be sought.

ACUPUNCTURE

A number of veterinarians have used acupuncture to treat muscular pain and other areas of pain and inflammation. The process should only be administered by veterinarians trained and/or certified in its use. This therapy continues to gain

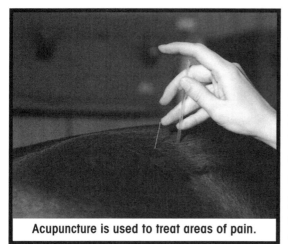

support, and its use in horses has increased. Acupuncture should not take the place of conventional therapies and complete lameness examinations. Appropriate case selection and application of acupuncture are important to maximize its utility, safety, and results.

Acupuncture is used to treat areas of pain.

The use of acupuncture to treat pain other than musculoskeletal in origin (i.e., colic) and specific diseases is increasing. At this time there is limited scientific information of the efficacy of treatments targeting problems other than pain management and musculoskeletal conditions. It is very important not to eliminate conventional medicine as part of the treatment of conditions due to underlying disease. Omission of conventional medical practice in such cases can be dangerous or fatal if such disease processes are not addressed with the more specific therapies available with conventional medicine.

OTHER THERAPIES

Veterinarians, owners, and trainers use a myriad of "other" therapies for all types of conditions in horses. Some of these therapies have received much more testimonial support than they have received scientific support. Nonetheless, there are a number of therapies used in a multitude of situations. For the veterinarian, a common and accepted position pertaining to such therapies is that they are welcome as long as they do not harm the animal. Opinions on the efficacy of such thera-pies will vary among veterinarians. Some therapies may be more helpful to the owner or trainer than to the horse. These therapies may have little scientific support and little physio-logic basis of effect. Despite this, a number of therapies are used that have no definable basis but appear to be helpful for unknown reasons. Indeed shock-wave therapy (see Chapter 8) might be categorized as one such therapy, with significant support of its efficacy despite a lack of understanding of why it is effective. Other therapies with significant support include magnets, which are believed to alter blood flow and perhaps reduce inflammation, and laser treatment, which is thought to increase the rates of healing of damaged tissue.

ACTH stimulation test — A test that is used to help diagnose a pituitary adenoma.

Adrenocorticotropic hormone — The hormone that tells the adrenal glands to release their products.

Allele — A genetic code for a trait inherited from the male or female of a breeding; usually, two alleles exist for each gene.

Anaphylaxis — A severe, potentially life-threatening reaction by the immune system to any foreign or new antigen introduced to the body.

Antigen — Anything that is recognized by the body as not part of its normal make-up.

Antimicrobial drug — An antibiotic.

AST (Aspartate aminotransferase) — A muscle and liver enzyme released from damage to either organ.

Bacterium — A specific type of bacteria.

Biphasic fever — A fever that "spikes," or peaks, twice a day.

Bowed tendon — An acute disruption of the fibers of the tendon that leads to bleeding and destabilization within the tendon and produces a "bowing" appearance of the tendon profile.

Bronchiolitis — Inflammation of the bronchioles (very deepest airways of the lung).

Bronchodilating agent — A medication that causes relaxation of the smooth muscle of the airway, allowing the airway to open.

Cardiovascular — Pertaining to the heart and the blood vessels.

Carpal joints — The series of joints in the front leg that begin at the top of the cannon bone and extend upward to the large radius.

Caslick's — A surgery used to close the vulvar lips of a mare to reduce the risk of developing infections of the reproductive tract.

Cecal-cecal — A type of intussusception in which the cecum of the large intestine telescopes into itself.

Cecal-colonic — A type of intussusception in which the cecum of the large intestine telescopes into the colon (large intestine proper).

Choke — Obstruction of the esophagus that causes salivation and nasal discharge with food in it.

Chronic obstructive pulmonary disease (COPD or heaves) — Chronic respiratory disease of the lower airways associated with hyper-reactivity of airways to allergens or irritants.

CK (Creatine kinase; also known as CPK, creatine phosphokinase) — A muscle enzyme released with muscle damage.

Coffin bone — The bone in the hoof; also called the third phalanx or P3.

Coffin joint — The joint between the bone in the hoof (coffin bone) and the middle pastern bone.

Coggins test — Blood test for antibody against equine infectious anemia virus.

Colic — Abdominal pain; this is not a diagnosis but is a clinical sign.

Colostral antibody — The antibody that exists within the colostrum of the mare.

Colostrum — A mare's first milk, rich in antibody.

Complementary therapy — A non-conventional therapy.

Corticosteroids — The types of steroids that are associated with significant anti-inflammatory effects (i.e., not the anabolic steroids that cause increases in muscle mass).

Creatine (phosphocreatine) — A mound in muscle that serves as a brief source of extra energy for work.

Cribbing — A stereotypical behavior in a horse that is manifested by biting down on a surface with the upper arcade of teeth and sucking air into the pharynx and esophagus.

Cyathostomes — The small strongyle parasites.

Deep flexor tendon — A tendon that runs along the back of the cannon bone that is just below the superficial flexor tendon and slightly closer to the back of the cannon bone.

Degenerative joint disease — A non-infectious progressive disorder of the weight bearing joints.

Dental arcade — The set of teeth.

Dentition — The structure and organization of the teeth.

Dermatitis — Inflammation of the skin.

Dermatophytosis — A fungal infection of the skin that usually causes circular areas of hair loss and can be transmitted to people.

Dexamethasone suppression test — A test that is used to help diagnose a pituitary adenoma.

Diurnal variation — Normal variation of a parameter throughout the period of the day.

DNA vaccination — Use of DNA introduction to cells to create the DNA product (a protein) that acts as an antigen to create the immune response against an organism, disease or other pathogen.

Dopamine agonist — A drug that has actions similar to dopamine.

Encephalomyelitis — Inflammation of the brain and spinal cord.

Encysted — Encapsulated form of life cycle where the organism or worm is dormant.

Epithelial — Tissue type that lines mucosal surfaces (surfaces of the body organs that open to the outside of the body).

Equine protozoal myeloencephalitis (EPM) — An infectious disease of the spinal cord associated with a protozoan parasite, particularly *Sarcocystis neurona*.

Equine viral arteritis (EVA) — A disease caused by a virus that may be associated with respiratory disease and abortion. The virus can be transmitted by venereal route from an asymptomatic carrier stallion to a broodmare.

Experimental challenge — An encounter of a pathogen by experimental administration (as in the testing of a vaccine efficacy).

Exertional myopathy — Muscle dysfunction and pain associated with inflammation that occurs in relation to exercise.

Extracorporeal — Outside the body.

Fetlock joint — The joint between the cannon bone and the first bone in the pastern.

Flaccid paralysis — Paralysis with weak and non-resilient muscles.

Float — The activity of filing down points and hooks that develop on a horse's teeth from its chewing motion.

Forage — The part of the horse's diet that includes long-stem and leafy vegetation, such as hay and grass.

Founder — The presence of rotation or sinking of the bone in the hoof in association with laminitis.

Genotype — A subtype of a serotype, primarily identified by DNA differences.

Glycogen storage disease — Muscle disease due to inappropriate storage of muscle glycogen (the preferred fuel for high-intensity exercise) associated with tying-up, muscle damage, and pain.

Heaves — A lay term that refers to chronic obstructive pulmonary disease or other lower airway hyper-responsiveness.

Heterozygous — The genetic information at each of two alleles for a gene is different, such as one normal and one abnormal.

Hock joints — The joints in the back leg that begin at the top of the cannon bone and extend upward to the large tibia.

Homozygous — The genetic information at each of two alleles for a gene is identical, such as two abnormal or two normal.

Hyaluronic acid — Lubricating component of joint fluid.

Hyperkalemic periodic paralysis (HYPP) — A genetic defect in a muscle sodium/potassium channel that causes episodic trembling and weakness.

Hypersensitivity reaction — An allergic type of reaction caused by prior exposure to an antigen.

Hypothyroidism — A disease state that causes inadequate function and/or secretion of the thyroid gland.

Immunoglobulins — Another word for antibody.

Immunotherapy — A type of therapy that focuses on priming or boosting the immune system against various infections.

Insect vector — An insect that acts as a mechanism of transferring a pathogen from one animal to another.

Intermediate host — An animal or other organism that harbors a pathogen and serves to help it develop further, then passes the developed stage to another animal.

Intestinal mucosal immunity — Local immune mechanisms along the lining of the intestine.

Intra-articular — Referring to delivery directly into a joint.

Intussusception — Movement of a piece of intestine into itself like the telescope that collapses down into itself by a thinner, narrower piece moving into a larger, wider piece.

Laminitis — Inflammation of the attachment of the hoof to the bone in the hoof, the laminae.

Larval migration — Traveling of the non-adult form of worms to areas of the body other than the intestine, usually through blood vessels.

LDH (Lactate Dehydrogenase) — A muscle and liver enzyme released from damage to either organ.

Legume — A family of plants that includes alfalfa and clover that provide higher protein and some minerals than non-leguminous plants.

Ligament — The soft tissue structure that attaches a bone to another bone.

Local immune response — The immune response at the site of introduction of the pathogen (such as the respiratory system).

Mastication — The act of chewing.

Maternal antibody — Antibody concentrated in the colostrum for passage to the foal by nursing.

Monovalent vaccine — A vaccine directed at only one disease.

Mucosa — The tissue lining a body organ that opens to the outside of the animal.

Multivalent vaccine — A vaccine directed against more than one disease (such as a "4-way" vaccine).

Muscle pigment — Similar to blood hemoglobin but called myoglobin and found in muscle as a small reservoir of muscle oxygen.

Natural challenge — An encounter of a pathogen naturally.

Navicular bone — A bone situated behind the coffin bone in the area of the heel of the foot; also known as the distal sesamoidean bone — the deep flexor tendon runs over the surface of it on its way to attach the coffin bone.

Non-legume — Not a legume.

Non-steroidal anti-inflammatory drugs (NSAIDs) — Anti-inflammatory drugs without steroidal activity and steroidal side effects; can affect intestines and kidneys with persistent use.

Occlusal — Pertaining to the surface of a tooth that contacts another tooth when biting or chewing.

Osteochondritis dissecans (OCD) — A developmental orthopedic disease that causes formation of cartilage flaps that flake off cartilage.

Osteoarthritis — Inflammation of the joints and bones.

Osteochondral — Pertaining to the bone and cartilage.

Pathogen — An organism or other entity capable of causing disease.

Pathologic — Causes pathology or damage or dysfunction of or to the body.

Parasitic pneumonia — Pneumonia due to inflammation caused by migration or other presence of a parasite in the lungs.

Pastern joint — The joint between the first bone in the pastern and the second bone in the pastern (middle pastern bone).

Percutaneous — Meaning "through the skin."

Pharmacotherapy — Therapy using medications.

Pituitary adenoma — A tumor of the pituitary gland that is relatively common in older horses and causes signs similar to those of diabetes in small animals.

Polysulfated glycosaminoglycans — Molecules that are associated with joint-fluid production and cartilage matrix and health.

Pruritic — Itchy.

Rain rot — An infection of the skin of a horse generally over its back and rump muscles that is caused by persistent exposure to wet environments and/or rain.

Renal — Pertaining to the kidneys.

Semimembranosus muscle — One of the muscles making up the "hamstring" of the horse.

Semitendinosus muscle — One of the muscles making up the "hamstring" of the horse.

Seroconversion — Conversion from the lack of a specific antibody in the blood to the presence of the antibody in the blood.

Serogroup — A subtype of a particular organism identified by differences in DNA and/or other characteristics.

Serologic response — The production of antibody in the blood in response to a pathogen; similar to the systemic immune response.

Serotonin antagonist — A drug that counteracts the actions of serotonin.

Serotype — A subtype of a particular serogroup identified by differences in DNA and/or other characteristics.

Spastic paralysis — Paralysis with spastic and tense muscles.

Steroidal anti-inflammatory drugs — Highly potent anti-inflammatory drugs with immunosuppressive effects and potential for suppression of body steroid production with long-term use.

Steroids — Referring to medications of the steroid class.

Stifle joint — The joint high in the hind leg that has the kneecap.

Subclinically affected — Infected with a pathogen but exhibiting no clinical signs of disease from it.

Superficial flexor tendon — The tendon that runs along the back of the cannon bone and is farthest away from the back of the cannon bone.

Suspensory ligament — A ligament that runs along the back of the cannon bone and lies closer to the cannon bone just below the deep flexor tendon.

Glossary

Systemic immune response — The immune response produced in the systemic circulation of the body.

Tendon — The soft tissue structure that attaches a muscle to a bone.

Transmammary — Transmission through the milk from the mare.

Tropism — Has an affinity for something.

Tying-up — An acute inflammation of muscle that can be associated with significant muscle damage and increases in levels of muscle enzymes in the blood.

Vagus nerve — The 10th nerve that innervates the head and is associated with control of autonomic (unconscious) control of many organs.

Vulva — The opening of the mare's reproductive tract.

Wobbler syndrome — A syndrome of a malpositioning or formation of the bones in the neck that causes compression of the spinal cord and nervous system deficits of the limbs.

Wolf tooth — The second premolar and often a small tooth in the horse.

INDEX

mosquitoes............22-23, 40-41, 50
MSM............79
muscle supplements............75
navicular disease............89, 95-96
nervous system conditions.....98-99
no rotation............42, 44
non-steroidal anti-inflammatory drugs............12, 84
nutrition............52, 54, 56, 58, 60, ...62-63, 65, 91, 100, 108, 111
oil............62, 74, 78, 100
onchocerca............48
parasite control............42, 50-51
pelleted feeds............52
physical therapy............80, 122
physiologic arrhythmia............100
pinworms............47, 51
pituitary adenoma (Cushing's Syndrome)............105
pituitary tumors............104
Potomac Horse Fever............28-29
protein............55-57, 59-62, 64-65, ...79, 100
PSGAGs............85-87
quarantine............7, 11, 16
rabies............17, 33-34
rain rot............99
regular foot care.........94, 108, 116
respiratory illness............92
ringworm............99
rotavirus............36-37
routine booster............10
selenium............56, 75, 79, 82, 93
shock-wave therapy......83, 89, 125
side effects............12, 15, 82, 84, ...102, 109
slow or annual rotation............44
small strongyles.........42-43, 45-46, ...51, 62
steroidal anti-inflammatory drugs............84
stomach worms............48
strangles............30-33, 92
strategic treatment............45
supplements............64-65, 74-80, ...82-83, 85-87, 110
tapeworms............43-46
targeted treatment............45
tetanus............14, 17, 24-26
threadworms............47
thyroid disease............75-76
ticks............49-50
trace-mineralized salt.......55-56, 61
tying-up............52, 80-82, 92-93
vaccinating the foal............13
vaccination............6-19, 21-25, 27, ...29-41, 92, 108, 111

Preventive Medicine sites on the Internet

Universities:
The Ohio State University:
http://www.prevmed.vet.ohio-state.edu
The University of Kentucky
http://www.uky.edu/Agriculture/VetScience
The University of Florida
http://www.vetmed.ufl.edu

Other Sources:
The Association of Equine Practitioners:
http://www.aaep.org/
The Horse:Your Guide to Equine Health Care magazine:
http://www.thehorse.com

Picture Credits

Anne M. Eberhardt, 7, 8.

CHAPTER 7
Anne M. Eberhardt, 65-72; Stephanie Church, 66, 68, 69.

CHAPTER 9
Dr. Nat White, 90; Anne M. Eberhardt, 97; Cheryl Manista, 98.

CHAPTER 11
Anne M. Eberhardt, 112, 115, 117.

CHAPTER 12
Anne M. Eberhardt, 123; Tom Hall, 124.

COVER PHOTO — ANNE M. EBERHARDT

About the Author

Bradford G. Bentz, VMD, MS, is a graduate of the University of Pennsylvania School of Veterinary Medicine. He received a master's degree in veterinary sciences at the University of Kentucky Maxwell H. Gluck Equine Research Center.

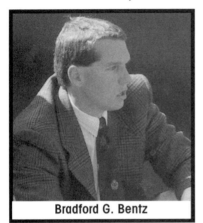

Bentz, who was born in Germany, is a Diplomate in Large Animal Internal Medicine with the American College of Veterinary Internal Medicine. He recently was certified in equine practice by the American Board of Veterinary Practitioners.

Bentz is an assistant professor in equine internal medicine at Oklahoma State University's College of Veterinary Medicine. He also maintains a private

Bradford G. Bentz

show horse practice.

Bentz has held numerous training and teaching positions and has served as a commission veterinarian for the Kentucky Racing Commission. He has prepared numerous papers for veterinary journals and has written for *The Horse: Your Guide to Equine Health Care*. He is the author of *Understanding Equine Neurological Disorders*, published in 2000 by Eclipse Press.

Bentz lives in Stillwater, Okla., with his wife, Patricia, and their son, Ian.